300 Healthy I

Everything you need to know about acquiring and maintaining healthy hair!

Natural, Relaxed, Color Treated and Loc'd

by

Saleemah Cartwright RN, BSN -Licensed Cosmetologist

Your hair is like your personal fingerprint. No one in this entire world has your hair but you. This is why it is so important to love your hair for what it is TODAY and have gratitude for what it will be tomorrow. Enjoy your own personal journey and love your hair for what it is now. If it is healthy, that's great. If it's damaged, love it anyway and start a healthy hair journey to get it where you want it to be. Enjoy each step of the way.
Saleemah Cartwright

TABLE OF CONTENTS

INTRO	3
THE BASICS	6
CLEANSING	12
DEEP CONDITIONING	17
MOISTURE / PROTEIN BALANCE	24
MOISTURIZING THE HAIR PROPERLY	28
DAILY CARE	34
STYLING / PROTECTING THE HAIR	38
NIGHTLY ROUTINE	43
USING HEAT SAFELY	44
HEALTHY SCALP	50
SHEDDING VS BREAKAGE	54
WEAVES / CHROCHET BRAIDS / BRAIDS	56
WIGS	61
NATURAL HAIR TIPS	65
CHEMICALLY TREATED HAIR	74
LOCS	82
TRANSITIONING OUT OF A RELAXER	92
COLOR TREATED HAIR	99
TRIMMING SPLIT ENDS	109
HAIR LOSS	114
HEALTH AND NUTRITION	121
EXERCISE AND HAIR GROWTH	124
HAIR ACCESSORIES	127
WARM AND FUZZY STUFF	132
PRODUCT RECOMMENDATIONS	134

INTRO

Insanity!

Albert Einstein defined it best- *Insanity*: "Doing the same thing over and over again and expecting different results."

My journey to healthy hair. Where do I begin! Most of the people who know me will tell you that I am a lover of healthy hair but it has been a bumpy road! I can honestly say that I have been through absolutely too many ups and downs when it came to my hair. Too many to count!

In the beginning, there were many more downs than ups. The reasons I went through so many trials and tribulations with my hair were utterly and completely my fault. Yes…..I take responsibility now but this wasn't always the case. I was the one to blame for my own hair troubles and the seemingly never ending setbacks. I have grown it, lost it, shaved it, damaged it, fried it, dyed it and started the cycle of damage all over again. I did this for years and years. I somehow expected my hair to magically grow long and healthy "one day". I didn't know how but I kept the faith. I thought that despite my unhealthy hair practices, my hair would one day be healthy and strong. Maybe a product or a magic pill would do it. Maybe if I find the perfect conditioner or ceramic flat iron. Maybe if I wear braids for a whole year to give my hair a rest, I would finally have my dream hair. My unhealthy hair practices didn't change for a long time but I still held on to hope. I now know what Albert Einstein meant when he defined insanity!

Early on, I was continuously searching for ways to achieve healthy hair but I just thought that it was a "genetic" thing. I thought that some folks were just plain lucky! Some were just born with hair that would "grow" and some weren't so fortunate. For a while, I thought that I was one of the unlucky individuals who couldn't grow hair. My hair would reach a certain length and then it would "stop growing". It seemed that my hair growth would be at a standstill and sometimes I my length would actually decrease. I now know that my hair was continuously growing from my scalp but I wasn't retaining length.

After much time passed, I just surrendered to the fact that I would never have hair flowing down my back without the assistance of a weave and I became dependent on them. I mean really dependent. I wouldn't go without one for more than a few weeks. I'm so embarrassed to say this but during my college days, I would wear that same darn sewin weave for the whole semester. Ewwwww. I did absolutely nothing to my real hair. Not even add oil to it. Needless to say, when I removed the sewin weave, my hair was in even worse shape. My hair would be matted, tangled with extreme breakage. I would always wonder………. why didn't my hair increase in length during those 3-4 months of wearing the weave? I was wearing a sewin weave to protect my hair………. my real hair should have grown out nicely right????? I still didn't get it.

I then thought back to when I was a small kid. I was looking through an old photo album at my grandmother's house. What did I see????? I saw a picture of myself from many years ago. I was probably 6 or 7 years of age. I had healthy, beautiful and unprocessed hair on my head! Thick, full and healthy. I totally forgot about the healthy hair that I had back then. It was a distant memory that I chose to forget for unknown reasons. I then went to the bathroom and looked in the mirror with much disappointment. My hair was extremely damaged. It was thin, lifeless and breaking due to my blond hair color and a relaxer. Many thoughts were running through my mind at that moment and IT FINALLY CLICKED!!!!

I realized that healthy hair is not a "genetic" thing that only the lucky ones could attain! My hair was completely unhealthy and it was totally my fault. I wasn't reaching my hair goals all because of me. This was when my healthy hair journey began. I began to read every book on healthy hair care that I could get my hands on and went to cosmetology school in 1998. Hair has always been my passion but now I had renewed excitement knowing that I could help myself and others!

After being discouraged for years with the whole "hair thing", I got my mojo back. I worked as a healthy hair cosmetologist for years. My husband and I later developed the healthy hair product line called Hydratherma Naturals while I worked as a registered hospice nurse. We later introduced the Hydratherma Naturals Hair Growth Plus Multivitamins to the market.

The idea of growing healthy hair can be challenging to some. It is really not as difficult as some would think. The only thing that is needed is a different mindset. Having accountability, knowledge of how to care for your hair, a consistent hair care regimen, great products and patience are all important components. It doesn't matter what hair type you have. You can acquire healthy hair.

I wrote this book to give practical knowledge on how you can better take care of your hair and reach your healthy hair goals. I also wanted to abolish unhealthy thoughts about not being able to achieve healthy hair. These practical tips can be added to your hair regimen no matter what your hair type. You can absolutely get your hair healthy again!

The Basics!

Here are some basic building blocks that will lay the foundation for this book.

1. **Understand the "basics" about hair.** Basic knowledge about hair is essential so that you can better care for your own hair. Hair issues may manifest in many different ways and the solutions to the problems may vary depending on the affected portion of the hair strand. Understanding hair vocabulary is very important so that you can attack hair problems and care for your hair properly. Here are some basic terms necessary to better care for your hair.

   Sebaceous gland -Produces an oily substance called *sebum*. *Sebum* moisturizes the scalp and hair.

   Hair follicle –A sac like structure that contains all of the components that create hair.

   Hair shaft -The hair you see, growing through pores located at the skin's surface.

   Cuticle -Encases the entire hair shaft. It is the hair's first line of defense. The *cuticle* is composed of up to 12 intertwined layers of dead *keratinized* cells.

   Cortex -The layer located directly within the hair cuticle. The *cortex* contains *melanin*, which are metabolized amino acids that produce hair color.

   Medulla -Located in the very center of the hair shaft. It is composed of round cells that are loosely connected to allow for air spaces.

Elasticity -The measure of how much the hair will stretch and return to a normal state.
Porosity -Your hair's ability to absorb moisture. It is broken down into three categories: low, normal and high.

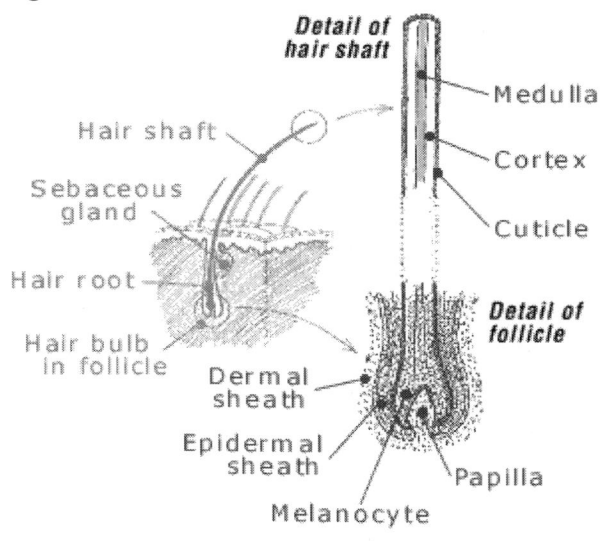

Detail of hair shaft
- Medulla
- Cortex
- Cuticle

Hair shaft
Sebaceous gland
Hair root
Hair bulb in follicle
Dermal sheath
Epidermal sheath
Papilla
Melanocyte
Detail of follicle

2. A.P.I E. of haircare. In nursing school, I learned the acronym A.P.I.E to problem solve. The same acronym can be used to solve hair issues.

   A- ASSESSMENT, P-PLANNING, I-IMPLEMENTATION and E-EVALUATION. This process is used in the health care field when dealing with health issues but it can also be utilized to solve hair issues.

   Assessment: First you have to know what your specific hair issue is. Is your hair too dry, too soft, breaking or experiencing slow growth? The first step is identifying what the problem is.

   Planning: Educate yourself on what the issues are and how to solve those issues. Develop a plan to get your hair healthy again. Your strategy may consist of things like deep conditioning your hair weekly, moisturizing twice a day, protective styling and /or trimming as needed. It is important to write down your plan so that you will easily be able to recall what you are going to implement.

Implementation: Work your plan. This can be the hard part so it is very important to stay consistent and dedicated. Some people may be super enthusiastic in the beginning but as time goes by, the enthusiasm may diminish. Because it this, I recommend that you take hair pictures monthly. This way you will be able to see your progress. Pictures don't lie. This will keep your motivation going and inspire you to keep moving forward.

Evaluation: This should be done after roughly 2-3 months. This is the time that you evaluate your plan. Is your plan working? Is your hair progressing as expected? Does you plan need to be slightly changed? This is the moment when you decide if you are on the right road or if you need to revise your plan. If revision is necessary, it's all good! Just move forward with a slightly different plan.

3. **If your hair is damaged, don't be in denial.** As mentioned previously, I made this mistake over and over. I was in some serious denial about my hair abuse and I needed to snap back into reality. Some people are in complete denial about their damaged hair. The first step to getting your hair healthy is to admit that there is an issue. Then……. do something about it.
4. **Hair Setbacks** – Hair setbacks impacts most of us. We may have some amazing hair growth goals in mind and something like heat damage or chemical damage will

wreak havoc on our hair. This can knock us back to square one after many years of attempting to achieve our healthy hair goals. I know that this is easier said than done but try not to be too disappointed if you are experiencing a hair setback. Try to view the situation in a "glass half full" way. It can be viewed as a learning experience that you can use to help someone else. It can also be viewed as a fresh start with a wonderful new hair journey ahead of you. This time, you will be well prepared and better equipped to reach your goals. It will also help you to enjoy your hair "TODAY". See next tip~

5. **Hair Envy-** I guess that it's normal to see someone with beautiful hair and say to yourself, "I want that hair". Some of us call others our hair idols. I have done this multiple times. It is probably better to call that person a "hair inspiration" instead. There is nothing wrong with looking at others for inspiration but not at the expense of tearing your hair down. Your hair is like your personal fingerprint. No one in this entire world has your hair but you. This is why it is so important to love your hair for what it is TODAY and have gratitude for what it will be tomorrow. Enjoy your own personal journey and love your hair for what it is now. If it is healthy, that's great. If it's damaged, love it anyway and start a healthy hair journey to get it where you want it to be. Enjoy every step of the way.

6. **Prevent damage before it starts.** There are many who have damaged hair and want to fix it after the damage is already done. In most cases, the damage is irreversible and the hair has to be cut or grown out. Try to completely avoid chemical damage, heat damage,

damage related to prolonged protective styles and damage related to increased manipulation to the hair. Once the damage has occurred, it is usually a done deal.

7. **Start a Journal-** Having a hair journal is an excellent method for writing down your thoughts, ideas and feelings about your hair. What are your hair goals and in what time frame do you want to achieve them? Do you desire thickness, length or both? Make these ideas clear to yourself.

8. **Realize that your hair can grow long and healthy no matter what the texture.** Kinky, wavy or straight. If your goal is to have long hair, thicken it up or just keep it healthy, you can absolutely do it! Why can't you?

9. **Hair growth rates.** On average, hair grows between ¼ to ½ inch per month. Hair growth rates can be boosted with the use of scalp massages, a healthy diet, exercise and vitamin supplementation. The use of Emu oil had been clinically proved to promote growth as well. Some individuals have naturally slower or faster growth rates but it is important to know that your hair continuously grows.

10. **Don't rely on your memory!** Take Hair Pictures! Take pictures of your hair every month and monitor your hair's progress. It is so exciting to see your hair transform from thin and lifeless to thick and beautiful right before your eyes! Sometimes you may not be able to tell the difference right away but if you look at a picture from a few months back, you will be better able to see a difference.

11. **Product Junkie-ism. Are you guilty of this?** Do you have 50 or more hair care products in your arsenal? If so, you are one of many product junkies out there. Some

people can't resist trying a new product and hair sampling clubs have contributed to this as well. This can be good if you are new to your healthy hair journey and you are trying to find products that work well for you. It can be detrimental if you run into multiple products that don't work well for your hair. My suggestion........Once you find great products that work for you, stick with it.

12. **Find a great stylist**. Some stylist focus more on hair 'styling' and less on hair 'health'. Find a stylist who specializes in healthy hair. If you stylist is "scissor happy", "heat happy" or "chemical happy", you will never see healthy results. When taking care of your hair at home, follow a straightforward hair regime that is advised by your stylist. A regimen that fits in well with your lifestyle. Finding a great hair stylist isn't too difficult these days. Just hop on Instagram and you will see many healthy hair stylists displaying their work.

CLEANSING

Cleansing your hair and scalp is one of the most vital steps of your hair care regimen. Keeping your scalp and hair clean will prepare it for absorption of your deep conditioners and moisturizers. A dirty scalp can lead to an accumulation of bacteria and fungus. This is the leading cause of scalp infections. An unhealthy scalp will unquestionably impede healthy hair growth.

13. **Keep your hair clean.** This may seem obvious to some but any buildup on the hair will prevent your moisturizing deep conditioners from penetrating the hair shaft. It will also prevent your daily moisturizers from penetrating and moisturizing your hair. This can result in severe dryness. If your hair is extremely dirty, deep cleanse / clarify, then deep condition and moisturize. Your deep conditioner and moisturizer will then be able to easily penetrate and do their jobs.

14. **If your hair feels dry, it may be a great time to cleanse.** If you have gone longer than 14 days without cleansing and your hair is feeling dry, cleansing may be necessary to boost the moisture levels. Moisturizing dirty hair religiously will not add moisture to your hair because the moisture is not able to penetrate past the dirt and buildup. The moisture will not be absorbed into the hair strand. This will result in more dryness. Cleanse your hair and start with a fresh clean slate. Please believe me........you will notice a huge difference☺

15. **It is best not to go longer than 14 days without cleansing and deep conditioning your hair.** Your hair has to be in its cleanest state to reap the benefits of your deep conditioning treatment. As mentioned previously, if your hair is not very clean, the deep conditioner or moisturizer will not penetrate the strand. If your hair feels dry after deep conditioning, it may not be clean enough. We suggest that you clarify and deep condition again.
16. **Keep your scalp clean and healthy.** Healthy hair begins with the scalp. Keeping your scalp clean will prevent infections and fungal growth which can impede hair growth. When cleansing the hair, apply the shampoo directly to your scalp and massage with your fingertips. Squeeze the remaining shampoo through the hair ends. Try not to scratch your scalp with your fingernails. This can be damaging to the scalp and can cause scalp infections.
17. **Use a moisturizing shampoo which adds natural oils back to the hair.** We know that some individuals are totally against the use of shampoo but cleansing the hair weekly will not cause any issues as long as your shampoo is gentle.
18. **Cleanse the hair in the shower.** This is an important step that should be taken to prevent tangles and unnecessary breakage. Apply the shampoo to the scalp, massage and squeeze through the hair ends. Piling the hair on the top of your head and rubbing vigorously will unquestionably cause tangles and this is what you want to avoid at all costs. Shampooing your hair in the shower will keep the hair flowing in one direction which will cut down on tangles.

19. **Clarify.** Don't be afraid to clarify your hair. Many hear the word clarify and they shutter with fear. The main worry is the fear of their hair feeling like straw! There are many gentle clarifying shampoos out there that will impart moisture and not strip the hair of its natural oils. Clarifying the hair is very important step in the moisturizing process. It is important to remove all dirt and buildup in the hair. You can even let your clarifier sit on the hair for a few minutes to remove excess buildup.
Product recommendation- Hydratherma Naturals Herbal Amino Clarifying Shampoo.
20. **Cleanse every 7-14 days-** Cleansing the hair weekly is optimal. As mentioned previously, I wouldn't recommend going longer than 14 days without cleansing and deep conditioning the hair. This will keep the hair and scalp super healthy. Remember ……..water is ultimate form of moisture so don't be afraid to use it as much as possible.
21. **Try co-washing.** Do you exercise daily and sweat up a storm during your workouts? Try co-washing your hair in between your weekly shampoos. This is a great way to refresh your hair and remove excess sweat. Just wet the hair and apply a small amount of conditioner to the hair (avoiding the scalp). Massage and let the conditioner sit for a few minutes and then rinse. Co-washing should not replace cleansing the hair because the co-washing method will not "cleanse" the hair and scalp properly. This can lead to serious buildup on the hair and scalp. It can also lead to excess bacterial growth on the scalp from the lack of cleansing. This is

why I recommend co-washing only between your weekly shampoos if needed.

22. **Oil Pre Poo.** This is an absolute life saver for those who have trouble retaining moisture. If you are suffering with severely dry hair, try an oil "prepoo". Before cleansing the hair, apply oil to the hair and scalp then massage. Leave the oil on the hair for a few minutes. Proceed to shampoo. This is a great way to retain moisture in the hair.
Product recommendation- Hydratherma Naturals Hair Growth Oil.

23. **Conditioner Pre Poo.** For a less dramatic effect, you can apply a moisturizing conditioner to your dry hair and let it sit for about 15 min to an hour prior to cleansing the hair with a moisturizing shampoo. This is a great way to boost moisture levels in your hair as well.

24. **If you are experiencing severe dryness, try going sulfate free.** I personally love sulfates and they do not negatively affect my hair at all. In fact, sulfates are the best cleansing agents and they actually cleanse the hair more effectively. Although it is a superb cleansing agent, some individuals are extremely sensitive to sulfates. It can cause dryness with some. Does this describe you? If so, the use of a sulfate free shampoo is a great alternative. Simply put, a sulfate free cleanser is a more gentle cleanser. It can remove dirt and buildup effectively without causing dryness.

25. **Cleanse using warm water.** I'm a hot water lover but not when it comes to my hair. Avoid using very hot water each time you shampoo. There is only 1 exception to this rule. See tip #26. Rinsing the hair with very hot water too frequently can cause the hair to

become overly porous. This will lead to dryness and the inability to hold moisture in the hair. It can also strip your hair of its natural oils produced by the scalp.

26. **Hot water rinsing exception.** Use hot water to cleanse the hair (very infrequently) only if your hair is loaded with buildup. If you use a lot of products in your hair and experience buildup a lot, using hot water every few weeks may be helpful. Hot water allows dirt and hair product buildup to be released from the hair cuticle as it expands. Always follow with a warm water rinse before deep conditioning. This will close the cuticle a bit.

27. **While cleansing your hair, be sure that you remove rings and jewelry that could snag the hair.** This will prevent unwarranted breakage and snags. I learned this the hard way. I would never remove my wedding ring under any circumstances but I then noticed that my ring would always have snagged pieces of hair on it after my shampoo………No Bueno! I now have a smooth wedding band and I have no problems. ☺

DEEP CONDITIONING

Please do not skip those deep conditioning treatments! They are extremely important for all hair types. If you can carve out an extra 10-15 minutes for your treatment, your hair will absolutely thank you in so many ways! Deep conditioning the hair with heat is crucial because it allows the treatment to penetrate into the hair strand. This will add moisture and/ or protein along the strand where it is needed the most.

28. **Deep condition every 7 -14 days.** Just as with cleansing your hair, we suggest that you do not go longer than 14 days without deep conditioning your hair. As mentioned previously, deep conditioning your hair is vital to your hair's health. That extra boost of protein and/ or moisture is absolutely necessary to keep your strands healthy and strong. It will also strengthen already weakened areas and prevent breakage. After you begin to deep condition regularly, you will notice a big difference in your hair's overall health.

29. **How long should you spend deep conditioning your hair per week?** Use heat to enhance your deep conditioning treatment but not for longer than 10 -15 minutes. Many people are under the impression that the longer they sit under the dryer, the more the conditioner will penetrate. This is not accurate. There is

no need to sit under the dryer for hours. After 15 minutes, no further conditioning will take place. 10-15 minutes is all that is necessary for expansion of the hair shaft and deep penetration of your treatment. The hair shaft will not expand any further after this time period. Any additional time spend under the dryer will not add any extra benefit. You may use a cordless heating cap or sit under a hood dryer to add heat. A great deep conditioning treatment is designed to penetrate the cortex layer of the hair strand and infuse moisture into it.

30. **No time for deep conditioning?** I'm sure that you can carve our 10-15 minutes to deep condition your hair per week but if you are one of those SUPER busy people out there, here is a great method that you can try. After cleansing, just apply your deep penetrating conditioner to your hair followed by a plastic cap at night before sleeping. Your own body heat will expand the cuticle layer. In the morning, comb through, rinse and style as usual.
Product recommendation- Hydratherma Naturals Moisture Boosting or the Amino Plus Protein Deep Conditioning Treatments.

31. **Don't have a hood dryer?** As mentioned earlier, deep condition with heat is always better because it allows the cuticle to open and absorb the deep conditioner easily. What if you don't have a hood dryer? You can try a cordless heating cap or try wrapping a warm towel around your head. You can also apply the deep treatment to your hair and wrap your head with saran wrap. Your own body heat will provide the heat.

32. **Deep conditioning extremely dry hair.** Here is a great tip that will enhance your deep conditioning experience! Add a little oil to the mix. After applying your deep conditioner, add a bit of oil to your hair ends. Cover with a plastic cap and deep condition with heat. Your hair will be very soft and moisturized! Great for the winter months as well! You have to try this method, you'll absolutely love it!

33. **By all means…..don't be extremely afraid of protein use.** Use protein deep treatments to strengthen your hair. Pleaseeeeeee……….don't be afraid of the use of protein. When you mention the word "PROTEIN", some individuals get deathly terrified! This anxiety typically stems from a previous traumatic experience with the use of a harsh protein treatment that left the hair hard, dry and brittle. Very harsh protein treatment may do this but these types of extremely intense treatments are not necessary. Your hair is 75% protein and adding a small amount of extra protein to your regimen is necessary. Protein will fill in the porous gaps along the hair shaft and strengthen the hair by penetrating the cortex and adding amino acids (simple proteins) to the portions of the hair strands that are weak.
Product recommendation – Amino Protein Deep Conditioning Treatment 2x per month

34. **Slippery conditioners RULE!** Conditioners with slip will make your life a lot easier. I personally love conditioners that give me a lot of slip! Tangles are easily removed resulting in less breakage. After deep conditioning, the comb will easily slide through the hair and tangles are easily removed. Most conditioners with slip contain silicone. Read more about cones -> Tip #36.

35. **Give hair steaming a try.** Some people unquestionably swear by it. Hair steaming may reduce breakage by increasing moisture retention. It is also known for stimulating growth by increasing blood flow to the scalp. Steaming may also help with dandruff by increasing the moisture levels in the scalp. If you haven't tried it, I suggest that you give it a try (at least once) and see if it is right for you.
36. **Silicones...Yes of No?** There are many online rumors stating that cones are awful for the hair. These online rumors promote unnecessary concern and is far from the truth. Don't be afraid to use cones in your hair. Studies have shown that silicones are easily removed with shampoo and will not "build up" on the hair. Cones protect the hair from heat and sun damage. Cones also provide "slip" in conditioners which will easily remove tangles. This will prevent breakage.
37. **Remove tangles easily!** The best way to remove tangles is to use a wide tooth comb or denman brush while the hair is saturated with deep conditioner (before rinsing). This will prevent breakage and will easily remove tangles. Trust me...... it will make your life easier. It will also save you a lot of time and energy on your wash day! Removing tangles on dry hair can be very damaging to the hair and can result in excessive breakage. Dry hair detangling is also more time consuming. Take it from me.....someone who has tried both methods (wet and dry detangling) on myself and my clients.
38. **Preventing breakage while detangling.** It is extremely important to comb your hair from the ends of the hair to the root while saturated with deep conditioner.

Working from the bottom up will decrease tangles and breakage. Take your time, listen to some great music and make it a relaxing experience. Rushing through this process will result in severe damage to your hair. The use of a large tooth comb is vital.

39. **Cold water rinses are awesome!** If you would like to add nice shine to your strands and increase moisture retention, you absolutely have to give this one a try! After rinsing the conditioner from your hair, let the final rinse be a cool rinse. This will allow the cuticle layer of the hair to tighten and close. This will lead to increased shine and moisture retention. If you are doing this in the shower, it will surely wake you up.

40. **Use a t-shirt to dry your hair instead of a towel.** Using a towel can cause frizz and can roughen the hair cuticle. It can also cause breakage by catching hairs in the woven fibers. It is definitely not a great idea to rub your hair vigorously with a towel. This will result in tangles galore! If your hair is loc'd be sure to use a t-shirt that is the same color as your hair. This will cut back on the appearance of lint in your locs.

41. **Microfiber hair towels ROCK!** These types of towels are great for all hair types. These towels are made from a super absorbent material woven from ultrafine microfibers. It is soft and less damaging to the hair. It also cuts the drying time in half because it is super absorbent.

42. **Don't exclusively use ONLY moisturizing deep treatments or ONLY protein deep treatments.** This is a mistake that I see many individuals make. Using strictly one or the other will cause hair damage and breakage as time passes. If you use moisturizing deep treatments

weekly, the hair will become overly moisturized and will break off. Breakage will occur because the hair will eventually become too soft. On the other end of the spectrum………if you strictly use protein treatments week after week, protein overload will occur. The hair will become too hard and will eventually break due to the lack of moisture. Keeping a balance is crucial. See tip #43

43. **Maintain a balance of moisture and protein in your hair while deep conditioning.** We will get more in depth with this topic a bit later in this book. One way to keep the hair in balance is to alternate moisture and protein deep conditioners every other week. Eventually, the hair will fall into a nice balance of moisture and protein. For example-> Week 1. Deep condition with a moisturizing deep conditioner. Week 2. Deep condition with a protein deep conditioning treatment. Continue to alternate every other week and your hair will eventually fall into balance. Using a harsh protein treatment is not at all necessary. A medium to mild protein treatment will suffice.
Product recommendations- Hydratherma Naturals Moisture Boosting Deep Conditioning Treatment & Amino Plus Protein Deep Conditioning Treatment.

44. **Does your hair still feel dry after deep conditioning?** This has happened to me in the past. I would cleanse and deep condition with high quality products. After deep conditioning, my hair would feel a bit dry. I realized why this was happening after a while. I was using a lot of brown gel at the time……Don't judge me…..This was in the 90's and everybody was using it. ☺ I had a lot of buildup on my hair and it wasn't totally

removed after cleansing (although I thought that it was). My moisturizing deep conditioner couldn't penetrate past the gel buildup even though I thought that it was totally removed. Looking back, I realized that the best bet for me would have been to clarify. If this has happened to you, there may be build up on your hair which does not allow penetration of your deep conditioning treatments. Try clarifying to remove any excess build up and then deep condition again. You will be able to tell a big difference once your hair is clean and able to absorb your deep conditioner effectively.

45. **Avoid shampoo / conditioner combo products.** It sounds great to have a shampoo and conditioner all in one bottle doesn't it? These types of products will not get the job done and I suggest that you avoid these types of products if you are serious about your hair. They will not cleanse effectively and they also will not provide optimal conditioning. There are many 2 in one products on the market. It is very important to deep condition the hair correctly. The shampoo / conditioner combos will not adequately deep condition your hair as it should.

MOISTURE / PROTEIN BALANCE

Did you know that you can 'over moisturize' your hair? Many people don't know this fact. Over moisturized hair can lead to breakage. Be sure that your hair is properly balanced with moisture and protein. This will greatly reduce breakage. Read on........

46. **Retention is the goal.** If your goal is to retain length, realize that unbalanced hair riddled with split ends will break just as fast as it grows. This is the reason many people will say "My hair will not grow". This is so far from the truth. Hair will continuously grow from the scalp daily but if the hair is breaking at the same rate that it is growing, the hair will appear not to have grown at all. In actuality, length is not being retained. There is a continuous cycle of growth and breakage that is occurring. This cycle will never end unless you become aware and stop the breakage. The goal is to let those inches add up by keeping the hair balanced with moisture and protein. Healthy ends will not break.

47. **This is MAJOR!** Maintain a great moisture and protein balance in the hair to prevent breakage. As mentioned previously, too much moisture will cause the hair to be very soft and will cause breakage. Using too much protein in your regimen will cause the hair to become very hard and brittle. This will also lead to breakage. Keeping a balance is very important to prevent breakage and promote length retention.

48. **How do you know which one your hair needs?** I get a lot of questions about how to get started with maintaining a great moisture /protein balance. How do you know which one your hair needs? After washing and deep conditioning your hair, look at a shed hair strand. Lightly pull the strand of hair. If your hair is spongy or gummy when it is wet, more protein is needed. If (when wet) it breaks right away when you pull (without elasticity) you need more moisture. If your hair is deficient of protein, I would suggest that you start your regimen with a protein treatment for the first couple of weeks. If your hair is moisture deficient, start with a moisturizing deep treatment. Just listen to your hair and it will tell you what it needs.
Product Recommendations- The Hydratherma Naturals Moisture Boosting Deep Conditioning Treatment and/or Amino Plus Protein Deep Conditioning Treatment will help get your hair into balance. Maintaining a nice moisture / protein balance is the key.

49. **Retaining length by balancing the hair throughout the week.** Weekly balancing of moisture and protein levels may not be enough for most. If your goal is to have longer and thicker hair, be sure that you take care of your hair ends everyday by keeping them balanced with moisture and protein daily. If your hair growth is ½ inch per month and your hair breaks at the same rate, the length and thickness of your hair will remain the same. If you stop the breakage at the ends, length will be retained. You can do this by giving your hair a boost of moisture and light protein daily to keep it balanced. Be sure that the protein that you add daily is very light so that protein overload will not occur.

Product recommendation for daily use- Hydratherma Naturals Protein Balance Leave In (adds light proteins to strengthen) and the Daily Moisturizing Growth Lotion (adds moisture and encourages growth). Daily use of our Protein Balance Leave In Conditioner and our Daily Moisturizing Growth Lotion along with sealing in moisture with our Hair Growth Oil will help you to maintain a nourishing balance during the week.

50. **Elasticity.** What is it all about? A great measure of healthy hair is normal elasticity. Hair elasticity measures how much the hair will stretch and return to a normal state. Hair in great shape will stretch 20%- 50% of its original length. It will then return to its normal shape. This occurs without breaking. If breakage occurs, the elasticity is low. Balancing the moisture and protein levels will help you to maintain healthy elasticity.

51. **Porous hair. What exactly is it?** Typically, overly porous hair is caused by chemical treatments, heat damage and over manipulation of the hair. Porosity varies from person to person. It is the ability of moisture to enter and exit the hair. Porous hair soaks up moisture quickly but loses it quickly as well. Overly porous hair can be more prone to breakage because of the spongy gaps along the hair strand. Those with porous hair tend to need a bit more protein in their hair regimen to fill in the porous gaps and strengthen the hair. After the porous gaps are filled moisture will better be retained as well.

52. **Maintain normal porosity.** A porous hair strand has a raised cuticle layer with gaps along the hair strand. Porous hair absorbs too much moisture which sounds great right? The problem is that the strand also leaks

out moisture. This prevents moisture retention. Overly porous hair tends to be chemically treated, damaged in some way, dull and dry looking. One way to normalize porosity is to stop the practice that is causing the damage and slightly increase the use of protein in your hair care regimen as noted in previous tip.

MOISTURIZING THE HAIR PROPERLY

Moisturizing the hair is an essential step that must be taken to get your hair on the road to health. Keeping the hair well moisturized is imperative because dry hair will break. This is a certainty. In this section, I will help you decide which types of products are best for moisturizing the hair and the best practical methods for moisturizing.

53. **Water based moisturizers.** Moisturizing with water based moisturizers is the best choice. If water is not listed as the first or 2nd ingredient on the ingredient list for your moisturizer, steer clear of it. Water based moisturizers will easily absorb into the hair strand and scalp. They will not cause buildup. Just think......water is the ultimate form of moisture so water based moisturizers would be the best choice to provide essential moisture. Steer clear of moisturizers containing mineral oil and petrolatum. More on this topic later. See tip 55

    Product recommendation- Hydratherma Naturals Daily Moisturizing Growth Lotion.

54. **Moisturizing with a purpose.** As we all know, keeping your hair moisturized and preventing breakage can be challenging. One great tip is to moisturize your hair immediately after the deep conditioning process. This is while the hair is still in its wet state. After washing and deep conditioning, rinse and section the hair in 4-8 sections. To each section, apply your moisturizer and

then seal in the moisture with oil. Style as usual. The next day you can moisturize and seal daily on your hair in its dry state to maintain a nice balance of moisture during the week. It is not necessary to wet the hair before moisturizing every single day. If you are experiencing dryness, this tip will help you a great deal.

55. **Avoid "moisturizers" containing mineral oil and petrolatum.** I know that many people are accustomed to these types of greases containing these heavy ingredients to oil our scalps when we were small children. As we know better, we have to do better. Moisturizers containing mineral oil and petrolatum will not add moisture to your hair in any way and will prevent your hair from being moisturized properly. Water based moisturizers that do not contain these two heavy ingredients will work best. These ingredients will not penetrate the hair strand and will only coat the hair.

56. **Moisturize Daily?** Is it really necessary? Well....It depends. Ideally, I would suggest that people add some sort of moisture to their hair on a daily basis. In some cases, it may not be absolutely required. As I mentioned previously.........Listen to your hair and it will tell you what it needs. There is no "one size fits all" regimen when it comes to how often you should moisturize or exactly how much product you may need to keep your strands moisturized. This will depend on your hair's porosity, thickness, length, level of damage and if it is chemically treated. Logically, it will vary from person to person. When you go to bed, run your fingers through your hair. Does it feel dry? If so, moisturize. If not, you may be able to skip that day. If unsure, moisturize ☺ I guess that it is better to be safe than

sorry. The main thing to remember is to add moisture consistently. This will increase elasticity and decrease breakage. It will also offset split ends.

57. **What should you focus on when you moisturize?** When moisturizing focus on the ends of your hair strands first and foremost. You can then work your way up to the root area. The ends of the hair strand tend to be the driest because it is the oldest. Give those ends that extra TLC because they need it the most.

58. **"Moisturize" and "Seal".** Moisturizing alone may not be enough for some individuals dealing with severely dry hair. To enhance the moisturizing process it is a great idea to moisturize with your water based moisturizer and seal in the moisture with oil. The oil will act as a sealant to hold the moisture in the hair. This is a surefire way to keep your hair super moisturized and soft. Product Recommendation- Hydratherma Naturals Daily Moisturizing Growth Lotion to moisturize and the Hair Growth Oil to seal in the moisture.

59. **Do not "over moisturize" your hair.** As mentioned previously, over moisturized hair will feel extremely soft and spongy when wet. It will have a wet cotton feel. Hair in this state will break without difficulty. If your hair is over moisturized, you will need to balance the moisture with protein. Once the hair is balanced, the breakage will stop and length / thickness will be obtained over time.

60. **Don't bother attempting to moisturize dirty hair.** Attempting to moisturize dirty hair is an enormous waste of time. Moisturizing hair that is kept clean is optimal. To moisturize effectively, the hair cannot be dirty with buildup. The goal is to have the moisture

penetrate the hair strand from the cuticle (outer layer) to the cortex (inner layer). If there is too much product buildup on the cuticle, the moisturizer will not be able to penetrate the shaft which will eventually lead to more dryness and breakage. It is so important to keep the hair clean. As mentioned previously, cleansing every 7 days is ideal. Going longer than 14 days without cleansing is never good.

61. **Avoid extremely heavy products (stylers / moisturizers etc.)** There are many products that are marketed as being moisturizer that are extremely heavy. Most of these products will cause heavy buildup which is difficult to remove and will not moisturize the hair. Many are not water based and will only give the hair a greasy / weighed down look.

62. **Hair oils do not moisturize the hair.** Oils are not moisturizers. Many try to use "hair oils" to moisturize the hair. Oil alone will not properly moisturize the hair. Oil should be used to seal in moisture "AFTER" moisturizing the hair. We suggest that you moisturize first with a water based moisturizer and then seal the moisture in with oil. Water based moisturizers penetrate the hair strand easier and moisturize better.

63. **Avoid the use of bad alcohols which can be extremely drying to the hair.** If you see the word alcohol in your product ingredient list, don't be alarmed at first. There are good alcohols and there are bad alcohols. The good alcohols are beneficial for hair. They add moisture by drawing water into the hair strand. Good Alcohols include Cetyl alcohol, Stearyl alcohol, Myristyl alcohol, Lauryl alcohol, Behenyl alcohol and Cetearyl alcohol. Bad Alcohols are usually the short chain alcohols and

are extremely drying. They are used to help products evaporate quickly. Bad alcohols include SD Alcohol 40, Ethanol, SD Alcohol, Propyl Propanol and Isopropyl.

64. **Moisturize more often in the winter.** Many individuals suffer from severely dry hair during the fall and winter months. During the winter months, the hair tends to become a bit drier. This is due to the cold temperatures and lack of outside humidity. If you notice extreme dryness, try moisturizing 2-3 times a day. This will increase moisture levels during the harsh winter months. You will notice a big difference. Don't forget to seal with oil ☺

65. **Moisturize more frequently in drier climates.** The summer time in the south east is very humid and the hair is in heaven (as far as moisture retention). On the west coast (desert areas), the climate is a lot drier. Keeping your moisture levels high can be a challenge but it can absolutely be done. People in dryer climates will have to moisturize a bit more often to keep the moisture levels where they should be. Try moisturizing 2 times a day and increase if necessary.

66. **Try a humidifier.** Using a humidifier may be a great idea if you have problems with severe dryness during the winter months. It will keep moisture in the air and will prevent hair dryness. It is also great for your skin. If you live in a dry climate, using a humidifier will benefit your hair throughout the entire year as well.

67. **Moisturizing the hair in humid climates.** If you are like me, you may have a love /hate relationship with humidity. I love the moisture that comes along with it for my hair but poofy hair can be a problem if that is not the look that I was initially going for. Although humidity

can cause frizzy / poofy hair, it can be very good when it comes to increasing the moisture levels in the hair. The frequency of moisturizing the hair in humid temperatures varies from person to person depending on the health and porosity of the hair. This may be daily for some and every 2-3 days for others. Feel your hair every morning and or night. If it feels dry, moisturize. It is just that simple.

68. **Don't forget about those edges!** Sometimes we are guilty of not giving the hairline the attention that it deserves. Remember that the hairs along hairline are the most fragile. Because of this, it is very important to moisturize the hairline a lot more often to prevent breakage. Give it the extra TLC that it needs. Massaging the scalp with moisturizers and oils (along the hairline) is a great way to promote growth and increase thickness in that area.

DAILY CARE

Education on daily hair care is absolutely crucial. When I worked as a stylist, I knew how important it was to educate my clients on how to care for their hair at home. With just a few missteps on their healthy hair journey, damage could result. This would knock them back to square one and they would come to me so that I could fix the damage. Sometimes I could fix things and at other times, the damage would be irreversible. Let's take a look at these daily hair care tips to prevent unnecessary breakage and unwanted setbacks.

69. **Check your product's PH.** You can do this with the use of PH strips which can be purchased at any pharmacy, drug store and online. The higher the PH, the higher the alkalinity. The lower the PH, the higher the acidity. A balanced PH for hair care products would be around 5. This is optimal. This is the same natural PH of the hair. You can simply dip your PH strip in your product and see what color appears. You will then match the color received with the color chart. This will determine the PH number. If the hair product is too alkaline, it will make the hair hard and brittle. If the PH is too acidic, the hair will be too mushy and soft. Either extreme will cause damage and breakage.

70. **Finger comb!** If you have to manipulate the hair while in its dry state, try finger combing instead of combing the hair on a daily basis. Honestly......Is combing the hair on a daily basis really necessary? The idea of not combing the hair everyday may be foreign to some but it will

actually prevent breakage because you are manipulating the hair a lot less. Less is best in this case.

71. **Watch those hangnails.** When you are manipulating the hair in any way, be sure that your nails are trimmed and filed. This goes for any manipulation such as detangling, setting the hair and cleansing. Hang nails will snag the hair and cause breakage.

72. **Avoid too much tension applied to the scalp.** Especially, along the hairline. This means that we have to be very careful with tight braids, sewin weaves and loc styles that pull the hairline very tightly. This will cause hair loss by damaging the hair follicle. Once the follicle is damaged, there is not much that the person can do except opt for hair replacement surgery.

73. **As mentioned previously, "Listen to your hair and it will let you know what it needs".** I know that I sound like a broken record with this quote but this is fundamental. This sound fairly simple but it can be difficult for some to understand what their hair is telling them daily. If your hair feels dry, increase your moisture levels. If it feels too soft and mushy, add more protein to your regimen. Balancing the moisture and protein levels in the hair is vital. This will decrease breakage significantly.

74. **Molecular roller sets.** Want those cute spirals without the use of direct heat? Try dry-setting the hair with the use of steam. Steam rollers will give the hair a nice smooth and conditioned set. This works best on relaxed or natural straight hair textures. It also works well on kinky hair textures that have been previously straightened with the flat iron. These types of rollers don't work well on kinky hair in its natural state.

75. **Alternate hair styles.** Many can fall into a hair rut and find themselves wearing the same hairstyle daily. Sometimes this can be severely damaging. Wearing a ponytail in the same area daily can cause breakage in the area where the ponytail lies. It can also cause weakness along the hairline with the constant pulling. Wearing cornrows daily can lead to a receding hairline as well. If wearing braids is your thing, that is fine. Just be sure to change your braid pattern from time to time. It is important to change things up to cause less stress to your hair follicles.
76. **Heat free pin curling at night.** Heat free curls are so easy to maintain. There is no need to use damaging heat on a daily basis. If you like to wear bouncy curls daily, you can just pin curl your hair at night. There are multiple methods used to pin curl the hair depending on the look that you are trying to achieve. Barrel, spiral and beach waves can all be achieved with the use of pin curls. There is no need to use heat daily or sleep in cumbersome rollers. Pin curl the hair at night. In the morning, just finger comb and go.
77. **Find a great stylist**. There are many DIYers (do it yourselfers) out there but there are some individuals who just plain don't want to do their own hair. That is completely understandable. Some people don't have the patience to deal with their hair and would rather pay someone else. Some may not have time to care for their hair correctly due to a hectic schedule with work and family. This not an excuse to walk around with unhealthy hair. Invest in a great stylist in your price range. Someone who cares about healthy hair and

someone who values your time. There are plenty of them out there.
78. **No teasing please.** This may go without saying but I thought that it was necessary to add. I have seen people tease their hair to achieve height. When I see people teasing their hair, I always cringe because I know that this causes damage to the hair cuticle. Tangles, split ends and breakage will be inevitable.

STYLING/ PROTECTING THE HAIR

Many styling techniques can be very harmful to the hair and can cause major hair setbacks. Things as simple as combing or brushing the hair too often can be detrimental. Here are some great ways to keep your hair protected from styling damage.

79. **Focus on "hair health" instead of "hair style".**
Yes…….There are many hairstyles that look amazing but can cause serious damage if worn on a consistent basis. Abusing the use of heat is a great example. Using heat too often can be extremely damaging. It is a great idea to give your hair a break from heat once in a while and opt for alternate styles which are less stressful to the hair.

80. **Roller setting to the rescue.** Roller sets are not as popular as they once were but they are making a comeback. Roller sets are very healthy for your hair. The absence of direct heat and the use of diffuse heat will always benefit your hair. It will increase moisture levels as well.

81. **Doobie Be Doooo!!!** If you are not fond of the tight roller set look, try a doobie. Roller set the hair with large rollers, dry under the hood dryer and the wrap the hair. This will loosen the curl and give you a smooth straight look with a lot of body.
Product recommendation: Hydratherma Naturals Foaming Sea Silk Curly Styler for roller setting the hair.

82. **Protective style your hair.** Protective styles are styles that keep your hair ends tucked away and protected

from the elements. This keeps your hair ends from drying out. This will give your hair a rest from heat and manipulation. The tucked away ends are moisturized and sealed with oil. Protective styles require no heat and do not require much manipulation of the hair. Your hair ends are the most fragile because they are the oldest. These styles protect the hair from air exposure and extreme cold / hot temps. There are so many fun options for protective style. Just have fun and be creative with it! I remember first hearing about protective styles from the beautiful model Wanakee in the 1990's. I knew what she said made sense because she had waist length relaxed hair. It was simply amazing. She definitely knew what she was talking about.

83. **Protective style options.** The options out there for protective styling are limitless! Change your protective style every so often to avoid damage. You do not want to wear the same protective style for extended periods of time because it may contribute to added stress to the hair follicle. (I.e. corn rows, sew-in weaves) Buns, braids, sewin weaves, pin curls, cornrows, french braids, twists, bantu knots, updos, lace fronts, french rolls, crochet braids or any other style variation that protect the hair ends. If your hair is very short, try twists, coils, corn rows, braids or wearing a wig.

84. **Choose healthy styling techniques-** Make the conscious choice to utilize styling techniques that are less damaging to the hair such as roller-sets, bantu knot set, twist or braid-outs (twisting or braiding the hair, allowing it to set and taking the twist or braids out for a free flowing style), loose ponytails, creative buns,

wrapping the hair, straw sets, molecular steam roller-sets or any other style that doesn't require direct heat.....be creative.

85. **Try not to leave your protective style in for very long periods of time.** As mentioned in this book's intro, I was one who would wear a sew-in weave for 4-5 months during my college days. The entire semester!!!! Yes.... I would wash my hair but that didn't prevent the breakage that I experienced. At the time of removal of the sewin, my hair would be matted and tangled. Extreme breakage would occur. Although 4-5 month is extremely risky, I wouldn't recommend wearing a protective style (i.e. sew-in / braids) for longer than 4-5 weeks max. I have included detailed info on sew-in weaves later in this book.

86. **The baggy technique.** This technique was extremely popular in the 1990's but it is still a great technique to keep your hair well moisturized and protected today. All you need is a plastic bag, your favorite moisturizer / oil and a drawstring ponytail that matches your real hair texture. Just place your hair into a ponytail, add moisturizer and seal in the moisture with oil. Roll your ponytail into a tight bun and cover your bun with a plastic bag. Cover the bag with your drawstring ponytail. The plastic bag will be completely covered. It's like giving your precious ends a natural spa treatment all day long.

87. **Get a protein treatment prior to wearing protective styles.** If you are looking to wear a protective style for an extended period of time (I.e. 4 weeks), it is a great idea to treat your hair with a protein treatment first. Maybe a few days before. This will strengthen your hair.

It will also prevent breakage at the time that you remove the protective style.

88. **Moisturize daily while protective styling.** This is of utmost importance. Many people protective style but forget to give their hair the TLC that it needs while it is being protected. When the protective style is removed the hair is dry and brittle. Breakage occurs and the person ends up where they started with no length being retained. This defeats the purpose of protective styling. If you are wearing crochet braids or a sew-in, two strand twists, coils or any type of protective style, be sure to moisturize your own hair every 1-2 days to keep your hair soft and well moisturized.
Product recommendation: Hydratherma Naturals Daily Moisturizing Growth Lotion

89. **Air drying!** Utilize air drying the hair instead of using a blow dryer. Air drying may take extra time but it is much better for the hair. If you don't have time to air dry and you are in a pinch, just use a hood dryer. The diffuse heat from a hood dryer is a safer alternative when compared to using a blow dryer.

90. **Don't forget to protect your hair from extreme weather temperatures.** Many people underestimate the damage that can be caused by extremely hot or cold weather temperatures. Sun damage can be very harsh on the hair. When going out in extreme temperatures, you can cover your hair with a cute hat or head wrap. You can also wear protective styles and use products that utilize UV protection. Keeping the hair properly moisturized also helps.

Product recommendation- Hydratherma Naturals Herbal Gloss Heat Protector to protect your hair from the harsh UV rays.

91. **Winter time / dry climates protective styling.** It is a great idea to protective style more frequently if you live in a very dry climatic zone. During the winter months, it is a great idea to protective style more often as well. It will help you to sustain higher moisture levels in the hair and this is very crucial if you are trying to retain length.

92. **Choose the right protective style.** When choosing the right protective style, avoid styles that do not let the hair breathe. An example of this is a sculptured type of style (using lots of gel or edge control) which last from one shampoo to the next. The quick weave is a great example of a style to absolutely avoid. These types of styles will not allow you to properly moisturize your hair daily. This will result in dryness and breakage.

93. **Don't overuse bristle brushes.** When I was a child, I remember hearing that brushing the hair daily will lead to hair growth. I tried this technique and it was an epic fail. It just resulted in breakage. Bristle brushes should only be used occasionally to smooth your edges if needed. These types of brushes should never to be used to brush the hair from root to tip. It can be awfully harmful to the cuticle.

NIGHTLY ROUTINE/ PROTECTING THE HAIR AT NIGHT
Protect those strands nightly! Going to sleep with your hair lose will definitely lead to damage and breakage. Here are some great hair tips that will keep your mane protected at night.

94. **Get rid of that cotton pillow case.** I would suggest that you invest in a satin or silk pillowcase. Cotton should be avoided because this material is absorbent and will soak up the moisture in your hair. This will result in severely dry hair. Satin and silk fabrics are smoother and will not cause friction. This means…….. fewer tangles and snags.
95. **Never sleep with your hair loose.** Sleeping with loose hair will lead to tangles galore! Before retiring to bed always be sure that your hair is tucked away in a protective style. I.e. Braids, pin curls, twists, wrapped, bun etc. This will prevent tangles and ultimately prevent breakage.
96. **Sleep with a silk or satin hair bonnet / scarf every night.** This will protect your hair as you sleep. If your significant other is not really feeling it, you can opt for a stylish bonnet. There are many online vendors selling lovely handmade bonnets that are actually cute. If you prefer to not cover your hair at night, be sure that you sleep on a satin or silk pillowcase.
97. **Moisturize before bed.** Moisturizing the hair before bed is the best time to do so. Apply the moisturizer to your hair, style your hair in a protective style and cover to protect. This will allow the moisture to soak in and penetrate the hair strand better. In the morning, your hair will be super soft and well moisturized. Just fluff and go.

USING HEAT SAFELY

Next to the use of chemicals, the improper use of heat is one of the leading causes of hair damage. Many people are unaware of the fact that heat damage can occur after just one application of heat. Once heat damage occurs, it is irreversible in most cases. There is not much that can be done except cut off the damaged portions. The best way to deal with heat damage is by completely avoiding it in the first place. Below are some great tips that can easily be applied to your hair care routine. Avoiding heat damage is vital because it can cause a major hair setback.

98. **Limit the use of daily heat.** The use of direct heat should be limited to 1 - 4 times per month. Using direct heat on a daily basis will lead to less moisture retention in the hair and will certainly result in brittle / porous hair. Remember brittle hair leads to breakage and breakage equals "no length retention". Thinness will result and eventually the hair will be extremely damaged, thin and lifeless.
99. **Limit blow drying to 1 -4 times per month.** If you are cleansing and deep conditioning weekly, blow drying your hair weekly should not cause serious damage. Be sure that your blow dryer is ceramic and not used on the highest setting. See tip 102.
100.   **Let's address "wet to dry" flat irons.** I have seen these particular flat irons sold a numerous retail markets. After shampooing and conditioning the hair, the hair is sectioned and the flat iron is used directly on wet hair. The hair dries after running the flat iron through the hair a few times. You can hear the hair

sizzle and crackle as the iron runs through the hair. This process is very dangerous. Please steer clear of these types of flat irons. The results may look amazing after the first use but after using this type of flat iron over time, severe damage is the consequence. Microscopic views of the hair strand show that the hair loses significantly more tensile strength and elasticity. It also causes severe dryness. It is healthier to bring out the trusty hair dryer and take the few extra minutes to blow dry your hair safely before flat ironing.

101. **Temperature setting.** I get this question all of the time. -> What temperature should I use to flat iron my hair? The amount of heat that the hair can take differs from person to person. If you are straightening your own hair for the very first time, start at a very low heat setting (i.e. 300-350 degrees). Then work your way up to higher temperatures after you see how your hair responds to the current setting. Increase the temperature of your flat iron only if needed. Starting at a very high temperature setting can result in immediate and irreversible damage.

102. **When using heat, be sure to only use Ceramic and or Tourmaline flat irons to straighten and or curl your hair.** This will cause less damage to your hair because ceramic / tourmaline technology heats the hair from the inside to the outside and not vice versa. Be sure that the flat iron that you purchase is solid ceramic/ tourmaline and not just ceramic / tourmaline plated. The top coating of ceramic plated flat irons will wear away quickly leaving you with hot spots along the surface of the iron.

103. **Throw away your traditional hot combs.** Hot combs can be extremely damaging because they contain hot spots along the surface. The temperature cannot be regulated and hot combs can burn the hair easily causing irreversible damage. There are some ceramic /electric hot combs available. This would be a better option.

104. Use ceramic / tourmaline blow dryers. Blow dryers are available using this technology as well. For our blow drying ladies and gents out there, just know that this is a much safer alternative in comparison to traditional blow dryers. Most traditional blow dryers blow the moisture "out" of the hair resulting in dryness. You can feel the difference in your hair's moisture levels after using a blow dryer with ceramic / tourmaline technology. As pointed out previously, ceramic / tourmaline heat is less damaging to the hair and more of the hair's moisture will be preserved.

105. **Diffusers are awesome!** A diffuser is a contraption that you can add to the end of your blow dryer to decrease the flow of direct heat. When blow drying the hair, a great way to minimize heat damage is to use one. It works amazingly well for wash and gos to speed up the drying process.

106. **Frizzy ends and the chase method.** Have you ever flat ironed your hair and still suffered from frizzy ends? This is more prevalent with kinky textures. Frizzy ends can be a problem if you desire a silky smooth press from root to tip. The chase method will smooth out those frizzy ends. The process consists of taking a section of hair and running a comb through your hair simultaneously behind the flat iron. This comb will

separate the hair strands which allows for a smoother press from root to tip. This method is less damaging because you will not have to pass the flat iron multiple time through your hair. This method will straighten frizzy ends easily.

Product recommendation: Hydratherma Naturals Flat Iron Chase Comb.

107. **Always use a heat protector to protect the hair from irreversible heat damage.** Never use any heat utensils without using a great heat protector. This not only goes for flat irons but for blow dryers as well. A great heat protector will act as a buffer between your hair and the direct heat.

108. **Using heat on dirty hair is a definite NO NO!** Heat should only be used on freshly cleansed hair. If not, you will be baking dirt and buildup in the hair strand causing extreme damage. Don't wait longer than 2 days after cleansing your hair to use any type of heat. Dirty hair will always burn faster leading to quick damage.

109. **Oil and flat ironing.** Using a very small amount of oil on the hair before flat ironing is very safe. Adding large amounts of oil to the hair before flat ironing will "fry" the hair. This is because oil heats up extremely fast and these higher levels of heat can be very damaging to hair. To use oil safely, just apply a few drops of oils to your entire head of hair and scalp before flat ironing. This will also keep the hair bouncy and will not give your hair a greasy / weighed down look.

110. **"Heat Trained Hair"** Many women with natural hair who wear their hair straight over 90% of the time may notice that their curl pattern has slightly loosened.

This is very noticeable when the hair is wet. A person who started out with a tight / kinky curl pattern may eventually end up with a looser wavy hair texture after the constant use of heat. This is commonly called "heat trained hair" but it is really a form of heat damage. If the person consistently wears their hair straight and is not experiencing breakage, it is nothing to worry about.

111. **How to get the bouncy look when using heat?** There are 2 types of presses that I have seen. A. Hair that is weighed down, greasy and doesn't move. B. Hair that is bouncy, moveable and shiny. The big difference is dependent on how the hair was prepped before styling. The amount of product and the type of product that is used will be the determining factor. Don't use excessive product (moisturizers, leave in conditioners and oils) before flat ironing the hair. This is a common mistake that I see regularly. If you want bouncy hair that moves, don't apply too many heavy moisturizers and oils to the hair prior to blow drying. All it takes is a pea sized amount of moisturizer, a few drops of oil and a few sprays of the heat protectant before blow drying and flat ironing the hair. I have seen many stylists soak the hair in heat protector prior to flat ironing each section of the hair. This is so not necessary and will result in limp hair for sure. My formula is 1- 1½ pea size amount of the Hydratherma Naturals Daily Moisturizing Growth Lotion, 3-4 drops of the Hair Growth Oil and about 4 sprays of the Herbal Gloss Heat Protector before blow drying the hair. This always results in soft, bouncy and moveable hair with lots of shine.

112. **Heat damage. Is it reversible?** This is one of the most frequent questions that I receive. When I get an

email from someone telling me their story about suffering from heat damage, my heart goes out to them. In most cases, I will have to tell them the bad news that it may not be reversed. It really depends on the severity of the damage. If the damage is not too severe, using a sulfate based shampoo and increasing the use of protein in your regimen may do the trick. If the damage is severe and the above trick doesn't restore the hair, the damaged ends may need to be clipped.

HEALTHY SCALP

In order to achieve health hair, the scalp has to be in tip top shape. An unhealthy scalp cannot produce healthy hair. Here are some practical tips to keep your scalp as healthy as possible.

113. **Perform scalp massages.** Scalp massages are absolutely fantastic! Massages increase blood flow to the scalp and increase the stream of nutrients reaching the hair follicles. This allows oxygen, nutrients, vitamin, minerals and proteins to nourish the hair root. This will help with thinning / weak areas and will contribute to healthy hair growth. Scalp massages can be performed 1-3 times a day. In addition to healthy hair growth, scalp massages have been clinically proven to reduce stress levels which can also aid in hair growth.
Product recommendation - Hydratherma Naturals Daily Moisturizing Growth Lotion, Hair Growth Oil and the Follicle Mist. The Daily Moisturizing Growth Lotion and the Hair Growth Oil both contain emu oil which has been clinically proven to promote growth.

114. **Hydrate the scalp by encouraging a slight increase in sebum production.** The purpose of sebum is to moisturize and protect the skin from viruses and bacteria. The production of sebum on the scalp can be boosted with the help of scalp massages, exercise and by drinking more water. It is also very important to keep the scalp clean. Without proper cleansing, excessive sebum will just sit on the scalp and becomes a magnet for bacteria and fungi. This can cause infection and create pimples on the scalp. This is what you absolutely would not want to happen.

115. **Prevent a dry itchy scalp with the use of hair oil.** A great tip to help with an itch scalp is to cleanse the hair and liberally apply hair oil directly to your scalp. Massage and then apply your deep conditioning treatment to the hair ends. Cover with a plastic cap and deep condition with heat for 10-15 minutes. Massage and then rinse. The added heat will allow the oil to penetrate the scalp. This method has been extremely helpful for many of my previous clients and current customers. If you have a dry / flaky scalp, give it a try.

116. **Moisturizing your scalp.** Another tip for dry scalp sufferers. Dry and itchy scalp sufferers will definitely benefit from the use of water based moisturizers as well. Applying a water based moisturizer to the scalp will allow for easy absorption. Mineral oil and petrolatum based moisturizers are not good for the scalp because these ingredients are not easily absorbed. They will cause buildup on the scalp and will not penetrate. Apply the water based moisturizer to your scalp and follow with hair oil to seal in the moisture. Apply to your scalp and massage. This can be done once a day.

117. **If scalp itching, dryness and dandruff is extremely severe, you can try the use of Sulfur.** Sulfur powder can be bought online and at pharmacies. You can mix the sulfur with your favorite oil (25% Sulphur and 75% oil) and apply the mixture to your scalp daily (and massage) to lessen scalp irritation and inflammation. Be careful with the use of Sulfur because it will discolor silver jewelry. It is also very smelly. Adding a bit of peppermint essential oil will not hurt.

Make sure that you do not have a Sulfur allergy before using.

118. **Give tea tree a try for your itchy scalp.** Tee tree oil is well known for its antiseptic properties and can be indeed helpful to eliminate an itchy scalp. You can add a few drops of tea tree essential oil to your carrier oil and apply directly to your scalp. Tea tree oil is also available in cleansing and conditioning products. Product recommendation- Scalp Soothing Shampoo Bar with tea tree and peppermint.

119. **Inspect your scalp monthly.** Many people don't take the time to do this but it is really important to notice any scalp changes as early as possible. If you notice any skin changes, discolorations, patches of hair loss or any signs of infection, contact your dermatologist right away.

120. **Try a Tricologist!** Have you heard of a Tricologist? Many individuals are completely unaware of the tricology field of study. A tricologist may be helpful for your scalp or hair loss issues. A trichologist is someone who specializes in hair loss problems such as hair breakage, itchy scalp and alopecia. They will be able to diagnose and treat most hair and scalp problems.

121. **Can your follicles actually be clogged?** Many say that the hair follicles can become obstructed with the use of certain products. This is not true. Contrary to popular belief, hair follicles cannot be "clogged" by using petrolatum based hair grease or any other product. Petrolatum based greases have no real benefit to the scalp and hair. It will only cause major build up on the scalp but it will not "clog" the follicles and stop

hair growth. The hair will continue to grow from the scalp as long as the follicles are still active. Greases will just prevent moisture retention and weigh the hair down. It will not stop the hair from growing from the scalp.

SHEDDING VS BREAKAGE

It's wash day and you are finished with your detangle session. You see your hair in your wide tooth comb and you start to panic. Is this shedding? Is this breakage? Is this normal? There is a big difference between shedding and breakage. The causes greatly differ. Some shedding is absolutely normal but excessive shedding is something that needs to be investigated. Breakage is typically caused by unhealthy hair practices which can easily be remedied with the tips mentioned throughout this book.

122. **Shedding vs Breakage...What is the difference?** It is extremely important know the difference between shedding and breakage. Shedding is typically normal but extreme breakage is not. One way to tell the difference is to examine a few hair strands in your comb. In order to do this you have to be extremely near sighted or have a magnifying glass nearby. What you are looking for is a small white bulb on the end of the hair strand (the follicle). If you see it, this would be considered shedding. If you do not see the small follicle on the end of the hair strand, this may be considered breakage.

123. **Don't be alarmed with normal shedding.** On average, shedding occurs at a rate of 70- 100 strands per day. Each follicle has its own growth cycle. Some individuals shed more and some individuals may shed a bit less hair daily. For this reason, normal shedding varies. If you are not combing your hair on a daily basis, you may think that excessive shedding is occurring when you eventually comb your hair on wash day. You may just be experiencing normal shedding from the

accumulation of hair during the week. If you notice a big change in normal shedding or if excessive shedding is occurring, consult your health care professional to see what may be causing it.

WEAVES / CROCHET BRAIDS / BRAIDS

Sewin weaves and braids can be a great way to protect the hair and promote length retention if done properly. These methods can also be a major cause of hair loss and breakage. I have personally seen many women experience severe alopecia resulting from the improper installation of extensions. Here are some simple dos and don'ts when it comes to braids, weaves and crochet braids.

124. **Weaves and braids can be great protective styles if done correctly.** If wearing a protective style in the form of braids or sew-in weaves, be sure not to ignore your own natural hair. As mentioned earlier, I was guilty of this very thing in my college days. I was wearing a sewin weave and completely ignored my real hair. I didn't moisturize properly (if at all) and didn't have a shampoo schedule. Deep conditioning wasn't done at all. My poor tresses suffered and it was a hard lesson to learn. My hair remained the same length throughout my college years and no length was retained although my hair was growing from my scalp. Breakage was a regular occurrence. Please don't make the same mistake that I made back then. Continue to cleanse and deep condition weekly. Moisturize and seal every 1-3 days. This will keep your real hair healthy and will prevent breakage at the time of removal. A great tip is to add diluted shampoo to a bottle and spray on the hair. You can also use applicator bottle to easily apply products to your real hair.

125. **Never leave a sewin weave in for longer than 4-5 weeks.** If your sewin or braids are left in for extended periods of time, matting will occur as the hair

naturally locks. Breakage will definitely occur at the time of removal. It will also be a nightmare dealing with all of the tangles.

126. **If you are wearing a sewin weave and your hair is in its natural state, don't overuse heat on your own hair.** I receive so many emails from women who experienced heat damage because they were wearing a weave but kept a little of their out to blend with the straight extensions. In order to get their naturally curly hair to blend, the use of daily heat was necessary. After the weave was removed, the heat damaged hair would not revert to its original curl pattern. Trying to blend your natural hair with weaves or wigs containing straight hair can cause extreme damage if heat is used daily to blend. If you are opting for the straight look try a full head sewin with none of your real hair exposed. If you must keep some of your hair exposed, only straighten your hair weekly after it has been cleansed and treated with your deep conditioning treatment. Be sure that the temperature of your flat iron is not too high as well.

127. **Opt for a sew-in weave that matches you own hair texture.** If your hair is curly, choose a curly weave. If your hair is kinky, go for a look with a kinky hair texture. This way, you will not have to fight with your ouw hair to blend with a texture that is not similar to yours. This will be a lot less damaging to your tresses.

128. **Human Hair vs Synthetic Hair.** If choosing from human hair or synthetic hair for braiding, choose human hair. Human hair will aid in retaining moisture. If you do decide to braid your hair with synthetic hair, be sure that your moisture game is on point. You have to

moisturize more frequently with the use of synthetic hair.

129. **Traditional micro braids (with added hair) are not protective styles.** Micro braids add a lot of tension to the hair roots because of the weight of the added hair. Micro braids with added hair can cause permanent hair loss especially along hairline. I have seen too many cases of this occurrence to count. If you like the look of micro braids, give "mini braids" a try. Mini braids are very small braids with no added hair. It is a really cute style that can be curled with rods, worn straight or can be crimped with a braid out or twist out. It is a lot less damaging to the hair follicles as well.

130. **Avoid tight braiding along the hairline because this can cause traction alopecia.** I know that many of you know this already but I still see many women suffering from traction alopecia (hair loss and damaged follicles) along the hair line from wearing tight cornrows, sewins and crochet braids. It really breaks my heart when I see this because traction alopecia is 100% preventable. In many cases, traction alopecia and can result in permanent / irreversible hair loss and the only solution is getting a hair transplant. If you notice light thinning along your hairline from wearing tight braids, stop while you are ahead.

131. **Take charge.** You may ask your stylist to not braid your hair tightly but they still may insist on it. They may state that they will comply but still braid too tight for your taste. If you are feeling any discomfort….by all means, let your stylist know right away. Don't just sit there and endure the pain. Your braided style or sewin weave should not be a painful

style to wear. Getting your hair braided should not be a painful experience at all. Comfort and healthy hair should be the priority of your stylist and if it is not, you should look for someone who is more in line with your hair goals.

132. **NEVER use hair glue.** There are not many people still using hair glue out there. I had to mention it because the use of hair glue will break the hair and cause hair loss from the root. It will also leave thick residue in the hair which is difficult to remove with shampoo. There is absolutely nothing good to say about putting this adhesive on your tresses. If your goal is to keep your hair healthy and strong, stay far away from this devil.

133. **The safest way to remove any form of braids after extended wear.** After removing a sewin weave, individual braids or crochet braids, be sure to comb through gently (with a light conditioner) and remove all shed hair before washing. Don't just unbraid and wash! You must comb through the hair with conditioner before washing. If this is not done, SEVERE matting will occur and cause severe tangling. In many cases the matted areas will have to be cut out and this can be devastating! I learned this the hard way when I wore braids for the first time in the early 90's. I just removed the braids and proceeded to shampoo my hair without combing to remove the shed hair. After deep conditioning and rinsing, I proceeded to detangle my hair and it took the whole day. I was so frustrated and I felt like cutting the tangles out. Some pieces I did have to cut. It was very upsetting.

134. **Protein Treatments**. After removing your sewin weave / braids, it is a great idea to give yourself a protein deep conditioning treatment to strengthen your hair. The hair may be very fragile because of the manipulation during the removal process. The protein will fill in the porous gaps and weak areas along the hair strand. This will provide strength to your hair.

WIGS

Wearing wigs can be a super fun way to change up your look. There are so many options when it comes to wigs now. You have regular mesh wigs, half wig, lace front wigs, human hair and synthetic hair wigs. Wigs are also available in many different textures from afro kinky to silky straight so you can definitely find something that matches your personality and your desired look. Here are some great tips to prevent breakage while wearing wigs.

135. **Why Not….Give a wig a try!** Wearing a wig is a great way to protect your hair and give your hair a break from styling, heat and manipulation. One mistake that I see women make is wearing a wig daily without taking a break. This may be really convenient but it can wreak havoc on your tresses. If you are in a situation in which you feel the need to wear a wig daily, remove it when you get home. Let your scalp breathe and give yourself a soothing scalp massage. If you wear the wig too frequently, it can cause breakage due to the constant friction of the wig on your real hair. I have seen many suffer from hair loss along the hairline due to wearing wigs that were too tight as well.

136. **Protecting your hair is crucial while wearing a wig.** It is not a good idea to just place the wig on loose hair at all. It's better to braid, cornrow or twist your hair under the wig. This will protect your tresses from unnecessary friction and tangles that are difficult to remove.

137. **While wearing a wig, be sure to wear a wig cap to further protect your natural hair.** After braiding /

twisting your hair and moisturizing/ sealing, wear a wig cap for even more protection. The goal is to prevent as much friction as possible.

138. **Try a half wig.** Half wigs are so much fun and look a lot more natural. The front of your hair will be left out and this will prevent breakage and stress along the hairline. It is super important to find a half wig that matches your true hair texture for natural blending. This way, you will not have to manipulate your own hair too much for blending. This is easy to do since wigs come in a wide variety of textures now.

139. **Don't place a wig wet hair.** This can create a breeding ground for bacteria and fungi. These organisms can cause serious scalp infections which you definitely want to avoid. Make sure that your hair is completely dry and well moisturized prior to placing on the wig.

140. **Don't sleep in wigs.** Sleeping in a wig is a definite NO NO! This will eventually cause extreme hair loss by rubbing against your hairline. It is better to remove the wig at night and perform scalp massages with a great moisturizer and / or hair oil.
Product recommendation- Hydratherma Naturals Daily Moisturizing Growth Lotion and the Hair Growth Oil.

141. **Comfortable clips.** Many wigs come with hair clips or combs to hold the wig in place. Be sure that the clips or combs that you are using are not adding extra stress to your hair and scalp. The combs should not be digging into your scalp and the clips should not be too tight. You do not want the added stress to your hair follicles. This will surely cause thinning, hair loss and scalp damage. If your clips are uncomfortable, remove

the clips or combs by cutting them out of the wig base and use bobby pins to hold the wig in place. Alternate the placement of the bobby pins to prevent stress in a particular area.

142. **Lace fronts / Moisturize your hair daily.** As mentioned previously, it is really important to remove your wig on a daily basis. With the popularity of lace front wigs, I have noticed that many people glue the wig on their heads and leave them there. I have also seen many people sew the wig on their head and leave it on for extended periods of time. This has to be the absolute worst because there is no way to moisturize and care for your hair on a daily basis.
A better idea would be to wear the lace front without the glue or to use tape that is easily removed at night. At night, moisturize your hair and seal in the moisture with oil. This will keep your hair and scalp really healthy.

143. **Plastic bag method for increased moisture.** This really aids in retaining moisture. If you are suffering from extreme dryness, you have to give this method a try. It consists of moisturizing the hair and covering the hair with a plastic cap before putting on the wig. The hair must be in its dry state and not wet before applying the plastic cap. You can even cover the plastic bag with a stocking cap to hold it in place and then put on the wig. This is like giving your hair a spa treatment all day long. This should only be done 1-2 times a week to avoid over moisturizing.

144. **Be sure that your wig fits properly.** A tight fitting wig can cause serious problems with hair growth along the hairline. It can limit the amount of blood circulating to the follicles in the hairline area which

would eventually impede growth. It can also cause serious breakage to the hair along with a terrible headache!

145. **Don't wear a wig that requires glue to secure it.** There are some amazing lace front wigs out there. Some are designed so well and it looks like the hair is actually growing from the scalp. The down side to lace front wigs is to get this flawless hairline, glue or tape has to be used to hold the lace down. The glue needs a special adhesive to remove it. This allows the wig to be worn for days at a time. This violates a few rules of wig wearing. 1. Not being able to remove the wig daily and 2. Not being able to moisturize the hair daily because the wig is not being removed. I have also seen hairline and extreme skin trauma due to adhesive use. It is better to use a clip to hold the lace wig in place (if possible). This will allow for you to remove the wig when you get home and moisturize your hair.

146. **Thinning hair with wig wear.** If you wear a wig on a daily basis, examine your hair and scalp frequently. If you observe subtle thinning and breakage, give the wig a break for a while. Pamper your hair and perform scalp massages to prevent further breakage and to promote growth. Don't overlook small indications of breakage and thinning.

NATURAL HAIR TIPS

Natural hair is hair that is completely unprocessed and is in its raw natural state. The hair is completely free of any chemical processes including straightening, texturizing, and hair color. Natural hair can be hair in its healthiest state but if not taken care of, it can become damaged as well. Here are some healthy hair tips to keep your natural hair in tip top shape.

147. **Utilize the L.O.C method especially if your hair tends to be dry and porous.** First, moisturize with your water based moisturizer, then seal with oil. This will lock the moisture into the hair strand and increase moisture levels. LOC acronym consist of- Liquid (water based leave-in conditioner and or moisturizer), Oil (to seal in the moisture) and Cream (typically your styler i.e. Curling cream). Product Recommendation- *Liquid:* Hydratherma Naturals Protein Balance Leave In Conditioner and or Daily Moisturizing Growth Lotion, *Oil:* Hydratherma Naturals Hair Growth Oil, *Cream:* Hydratherma Naturals Aloe Curl Enhancing Twisting Cream. This combination will keep your hair super soft and well moisturized.

148. **Excess product usage.** I have noticed that many naturalistas tend to overdo it when it comes to the amounts of products used. This is especially true for conditioners, moisturizers and stylers. With most high quality products, a little goes a long way so there is no need to add globs and globs of conditioner and moisturizers to your hair. This will also give the hair a greasy look. If you are unfamiliar with a product, just section your hair and apply a small amount per section

first. Then, work your way up and use more only if necessary. This will also save money since you are not running through so many products on a weekly basis.

149. **Manipulate natural hair very little when in its dry state.** Finger combing is best when it comes to manipulating dry natural hair. The best time to comb the hair is when it is soaking wet and saturated with deep conditioner. This way, breakage will be minimized. A great deep conditioner will give the hair enough slip and moisture to allow for easy detangling. There is absolutely no need to comb dry hair on a daily basis because it will definitely lead to breakage and thinning.

150. **Handle your hair with care.** As mentioned in the previous tip, low manipulation is key! This is especially true when the hair is in its dry state. Try to manipulate the hair as little as possible on a daily basis and leave it alone. Most styling should consist of finger combing and fluffing the hair. Combing, brushing and constant detangling of the hair should be minimized to avoid breakage.

151. **Detangling Natural Hair.** It is very important to section natural hair is small sections while detangling. At least 6-8 sections should be good. The smaller the section, the better. When detangling the hair, work from the ends upward with your wide tooth comb or denman brush. This is key to preventing breakage. Attempting to detangle the hair from the scalp downward is a surefire way to increase breakage. Proceed to detangle from the hair ends upward in 1-2 inch increments until all of the hair is completely detangled. This is best done when your hair is saturated with deep conditioner.

152. **Minimize single strand knots (SSKs) which can cause breakage.** Those darn single strand knots!!! If your hair is kinky, you know exactly what those pesky knots are. SSKs typically occur with tightly curled and kinky hair textures. They are tiny knots that form on a single strand of the hair due to the hair curling on itself. These knots can cause breakage while combing and detangling. The hair will typically break right above the knot. This is also a problem that cannot be completely eliminated but it can be minimized.

A few tips to minimize those irritating single strand knots->

Preventing tangles - This helps a great deal. Keeping the hair detangled will prevent knots from forming. As mentioned previously, it is a great idea not to comb your hair daily. Just lightly detangle with your fingers because it is less damaging. Be sure to remove all shed hairs as well. While shampooing and deep conditioning, it is best to work in sections to prevent tangles and it is also best to shampoo the hair in the shower.

Trim the hair - Sometimes split ends can contribute to single strand knots. This is because the frayed ends can become intertwined with each other and form knots easily. Healthy ends are less likely to do this.

Maintain a nice moisture / protein balance - This will keep your hair in an overall healthier state. Hair that is well balanced will experience less knots.

Oil rinse – Oil rinses work extremely well because it adds extra lubrication on the hair ends. This is helpful when it comes to preventing SSKs. I have used this method and it works like a charm. After cleansing, deep conditioning and detangling the hair, apply the oil from root to tip. Leave the oil on your hair for a few minutes and work it into your strands with your fingers. Squeeze through then rinse. You will absolutely love the way your hair feels!

Search and destroy – This method is only for those with extreme patience because it takes a great deal of time. It consists of sectioning the hair and going through each section (strand by strand) looking for the knots. You can clip them or use a small pin to unravel the knot.

Shampoo the scalp and manipulate the hair very little while washing - I suggest that you apply the shampoo directly to your scalp, massage and squeeze through the hair ends. This will prevent tangles resulting in less single strand knots. Product recommendation-> Apply a dime to a quarter size amount of the Hydratherma Naturals Moisture Boosting Shampoo to your scalp and squeeze through to the hair ends. Shampooing the hair in sections will help with longer lengths.

Protect your hair at night - Braiding or twisting the hair before retiring to bed is particularly important when it comes to preventing SSKs. You do not want your hair loose while sleeping because this cause extreme tangling and even more SSKs. Always sleep with silk or satin scarf or bonnet.

153. **Are you a straight natural?** A straight natural is a term used to describe a person who has naturally kinky hair and wears their hair straight most of the time. It is very possible to have healthy heat treated hair and not suffer from heat damage. It is important for straight naturals keep up with their protein treatments regularly to prevent breakage and

strengthen the hair. Trims may be needed a bit more frequently in comparison to those who do not use heat at all.

154. **Avoid heat damage as a straight natural.** Try straightening your hair no more than 2 times per month. It really hurts me when I receive an email from someone stating that they have experienced heat damage and their hair is no longer reverting back to its curly / kinky state. In many cases, the hair will never revert back and remains straight. Heat damage can occur over time or after only one application of heat. Heat damage will permanently alter the texture of natural curls and coils making the hair straight and lifeless. In some cases, the curls may loosen and bounce back but in most cases, the damage is irreversible.

155. **Already suffering from heat damage?** Now what? If the damage is not too severe, the use of sulfate shampoos and protein treatments may give the curls a boost as mentioned in one of my previous tips. You can shampoo your hair 1-2 times a week with a sulfate based shampoo and then deep condition with a protein based deep conditioning treatment. You can do this for 3 weeks. If your hair has not reverted to its curly state in this time period, there is a strong chance that your hair is permanently damaged. If the heat damage is too harsh, the damaged ends must be grown out and ultimately clipped. It can be very difficult to style your hair with 2 extremely different textures. If you don't want to cut your damaged ends off all at once, you can wear very curly styles to hide the texture differences. Rod sets or straw sets may be your best friend during

this transition time. Two strand twists with rods on the hair ends (to set the curl) work great as well.

156. **Know your hair texture.** This may seem obvious but it is very important. Knowing your hair texture will allow you to better care for your hair. This is because hair care needs are slightly different for each hair type. A person with a very kinky hair texture will tend to have more issues with dryness. Kinky hair textures are very coily and the natural / moisturizing oils produced by the scalp cannot move from the scalp to the hair ends easily. This person will have to moisturize their ends more frequently to retain moisture. A person with a looser curl pattern or straight hair may have to moisturize a bit less often because the scalp sebum can easily move down the hair strand from root to tip. This is why knowing your hair type will help you to better care for your hair.

157. **If your hair is natural, please don't ignore those split ends.** Although split ends aren't as noticeable on natural hair, you still want to clip them so that you hair will be able to achieve its maximum length and thickness. Ignoring split ends is dangerous because split ends will eventually break off. Those with natural hair can use the twist and clip technique for split end trimming. We will go into more details on this subject in the trimming section.

158. **Making your curls pop.** The key to making your curls pop is proper moisture retention and hydration techniques. This makes a huge difference. Make sure that your curls are thoroughly moisturized with water based moisturizers. Also, be sure to use a high quality curl definer loaded with moisturizing ingredients and

botanical extracts. Only hydrated curls will pop! We suggest moisturizing your curls with your water based moisturizer while your hair is soaking wet instead of dry. Moisturizing your curls while wet will hydrate your curls better.

Product recommendations-> Hydratherma Naturals Aloe Curl Enhancing Twisting Cream and the Daily Moisturizing Growth Lotion.

159. **Shrinkage and styling.** Shrinkage...You either love it or hate it. Those may hate it because it doesn't really display their true length. I definitely understand. You have been growing your hair out for years and you wanna show off that length but it seems to be only a few inches long. You know that it is really 4 times that length. Those may love it because it is a true sign of healthy hair. If you pull the hair and it springs right back up, you know that your hair is healthy and strong. It's better than having heat damaged hair right??? As far as styling the hair goes->……..If you really want your hair to appear longer, I suggest that you go for braid outs instead of twist outs. Braid outs will elongate the hair a bit more and the larger the braid the more the hair will stretch.

160. **How to elongate your natural curls with a wash and go.** I get this question a lot. Many want to know how they can cut back on some of the shrinkage that they are experiencing. Elongation of curls comes from styling techniques and not necessarily hair products. Here is great technique to elongate your curls -> A. Cleanse and condition. B. Section your hair off in 4-6 sections. C. Moisturize and seal. D. Apply your styler to each section soaking wet hair liberally. E. Define

your curls with your finger or with denman brush. F. Add water to the hair again (just a bit) and sit under hood dryer until 70% dry. G. Section your hair and go through each section with a hair dryer (diffuser attached) while stretching the hair and holding it taut. Do this to each section until completely dry. This is a technique that will actually lengthen the curls.

161. **Big Hair Don't Care!** I absolutely LOVEEEEEE big hair! The bigger the better. There is nothing like confidently walking into a room with all of that big hair and all eyes are on you! There is something really funky and dope about that! If you want great big hair, a great technique is to lightly blow the hair out a bit before braiding or twisting the hair. This will lengthen the hair and give you that big hair that you desire.

162. **Minimizing the frizz.** Here is a great trick that works very well to cut down on frizz. Try "cool rinses". After deep conditioning the hair and rinsing out the deep conditioner, let the final rinse be a cool rinse. Rinse the hair for about 20 -30 seconds with very cold water. The colder, the better. Cool rinses will cause the cuticle to tighten and the hair strand will form a more defined curl. Give it a try it really works. It may be slightly uncomfortable but it is really worth the brief chill!

163. **Preventing reversion with your curly look (twist outs, braid outs, bantu curls etc.)** Let's face it. You really don't want to spend hours prepping your hair for the bomb twist-out and go out in the humidity just to watch your hair go POOF within minutes! The reality is....... you will experience some reversion in the humidity. This is something that can't be totally avoided

but it can be minimized. There are 2 things that will prevent some of the reversion that you will experience in the humidity. 1. -Using an oil (to prevent much absorption of the environmental moisture in the air) and 2. -a great "styler" (to provide hold). This product combo will really help! If you want your style to last longer, be sure to prep your braid outs / twist outs on wet hair for a more defined and long lasting look. Product recommendations-> Hydratherma Naturals Hair Growth Oil and the Aloe Curl Enhancing Twisting Cream.

CHEMICALLY TREATED HAIR

Chemically treated hair can be healthy. The key is taking those extra steps to keep it healthy and balanced. If your chemically treated hair is imbalanced with moisture and protein, serious damage can occur resulting in breakage. Here are some great tips to keep your color treated, relaxed or texturized hair in amazing shape. Breakage and increased porosity are major challenges faced by those who are chemically processed. With the right regimen, breakage can be tremendously reduced.

164. **Is chemically treated hair more fragile?** Since relaxed, color treated and texturized hair is chemically processed, it is much more fragile and porous. The natural bonds in the hair are broken and it is more susceptible to breakage. This is why I suggest using low or no direct heat styling. Using too much heat on chemically treated hair will wear away the cuticle layer of the hair and cause serious damage and breakage. The hair will become very brittle. I have experienced this first hand when I was in college. I went through part of the year using daily heat on my relaxed hair. I started out with bra strap length hair and ended up with shoulder length hair within a few months. My hair was also so thin that you could actually see through it easily. I ended up having to wear a weave because it was so thin and there was absolutely nothing that I could do with it except cut it off. I didn't want to go the cutting route so I opted for a weave until my hair grew back.

If you are using heat on a daily basis, try giving your hair a much needed break. You will notice a huge difference within a few months. There are many styles that can be done with low or no heat such as braid outs, bantu curls, roller sets, flexirod sets, rod sets and wrapping the hair at night. If you are completely unfamiliar with these types of styles, just go to YouTube and check out some tutorials. Your hair will absolutely love you for it.

165. **Protective style often to reduce the amount of heat used.** If your hair is chemically treated, protective styling should be your best friend. Bunning, updos and braid styles are great "go to" styles. Be sure to moisturize and seal with oil before protective styling. This is like giving your hair a spa day!

166. **Nightly routine for chemically treated hair.** If your hair is relaxed, try pin curling your hair at night. This is a great alternative to using heat and depending on the pin curling technique used; you can get anything from deep waves to tight spiral curls. It will also save you valuable time in the morning because all you have to do is lightly finger comb and go. Just think, you don't have to spend the extra time curling your hair in the morning and we all know that every minute counts when you are getting ready for work.

167. **Seek a professional.** Many people feel very confident applying chemicals to their hair but this doesn't necessarily mean that it is the safe route to go. I know many who feel extremely comfortable relaxing or coloring their own hair but their hair doesn't actually look healthy at all. It is awfully difficult to not process previously relaxed hair with the relaxer / texturizer cream. This will surely result in extreme damage and

over processed hair. If you are not confident with chemical processing, please seek a professional with loads of experience.

168. **There is no need to relax your hair bone straight.** This will definitely result in hair with no elasticity and hair without elasticity will certainly break off. After the relaxer is applied, there should still be some sort of wave left. Relax the hair only about 70-80%. Relaxing this way will be less damaging and it will also give the hair more body / fullness.

169. **Never use a "super" relaxer.** Relaxers typically come in a mild, regular and super. Using a super relaxer is simply not necessary for any hair type. Even the most kinky textures wouldn't need it. Getting the hair straight is more about the method of application and not about the relaxer strength. Most hair textures can use a mild relaxer and get nice results by working the relaxer into the hair properly.

170. **Don't believe the No-Lye Lie.** Contrary to popular belief using a lye based sodium hydroxide relaxer is better for the hair when compared to a no lye relaxer ......hands down. A lye relaxer is the better choice because no lye relaxers use calcium hydroxide. Calcium Hydroxide leaves a calcium deposit on the hair. This calcium deposit will coat the hair shaft and will prevent moisture from entering the hair properly. This will eventually lead to extreme dryness, split ends and breakage over time. No matter how much you attempt to moisturize the hair, it will never be properly moisturized because of the calcium deposits. Sodium Hydroxide (lye) relaxers will not do this. Lye will actually leave the hair shinier because it closes the cuticles

properly. Hair that is treated with lye will also be easier to moisturize.

I can tell right away if someone is using a no lye relaxer because the hair will have a dull look and breakage is usually evident.

171. **Avoid box relaxer kits.** To all of you "do it yourselfers", PLEASE avoid box relaxer kits by any means necessary. These relaxer kits will most likely contain the ingredient Calcium Hydroxide (no lye) and it should definitely be avoided like the plague.

172. **Relax the hair no less than every 8 weeks.** I remember when I was in cosmetology school in the 1990's. We were taught to give relaxer touchups every 6 weeks. Some of my friends relaxed every 4 weeks! Now that I am a lot more educated on healthy hair practices, I look back on this teaching and cringe. If you can go longer than 8 weeks without experiencing breakage, go for it!

173. **If your hair is already damaged, do not relax your hair.** I have seen many stylists relax their client's hair when it was obviously severely damaged. Some stylists are more concerned with taking their clients' money and less concerned with healthy hair. If your stylist is interested in the health of your hair, relaxing damaged hair is something that they simply would not do. This will result in severe damage, thinning and hair loss. It is better to treat the hair first with a series of protein treatments (to strengthen the hair) and then revaluate at a later time.

174. **If you are experiencing scalp problems, do not relax.** This should go without saying but some people still apply chemicals to their hair while suffering from

scalp issues. You absolutely do not want to apply any chemicals to a damaged scalp because this will result in severe injury to the scalp and hair follicles. It could result in permanent scalp damage and irreversible hair loss. In this case, I would suggest that you consult a dermatologist and resolve the scalp issue first before applying chemicals.

175. **Relax only new growth.** Do not apply relaxer to already processed hair. As mentioned previously, it is difficult to not overlap and apply the relaxer to previously relaxed hair if you are doing your own relaxer. This is why we suggest seeking a professional who specializes in healthy hair. Overlapping will cause damage in the long run.

176. **Try relaxer stretching.** Relaxer stretching consists of relaxing the hair less often. The amount of time differs from person to person but it generally involves relaxing the hair every 3-12 months. This will prevent over processing the hair. Over processed hair will undoubtedly break. Relaxer stretching needs to be done with care because severe breakage can occur if done incorrectly. Some people can go 3 months before they begin to experience breakage at the line of demarcation (point along the hair strand where the relaxed hair ends and the natural hair begins). It is also the weakest area along the hair strand. Some people can go up to 12 months before they relax again with no difficulty. I noticed that kinky hair textures cannot relaxer stretch as long as those who have looser curl patterns. If you decide to relaxer stretch, be sure to watch your hair closely and look for any breakage that

may occur. See next hair tip to learn how to cut down on breakage while relaxer stretching.

177. **If you decide to relaxer stretch, it is extremely crucial to keep your new growth exceptionally moisturized.** Increasing the moisture level of your new growth is a very important step that needs to be taken to avoid breakage. If your hair is not well moisturized, it will break at the line of demarcation. The breakage will only intensify as time passes if the hair is not properly moisturized. This will definitely cause a terrible hair setback and defeats the purpose of relaxer stretching. Just take a few extra minutes a day to correctly moisturize and seal your new growth. It will make a huge difference in preventing breakage!
Product recommendation- Hydratherma Naturals Daily Moisturizing Growth Lotion to moisturize and the Hair Growth Oil to seal in the moisture.

178. **If you decide to relax your own hair, relax your hair in sections to avoid over or under processing.** This takes a bit more time but the health of your hair is certainly worth it. This can be done by sectioning the hair in two sections (parting the hair from ear to ear or parting your hair down the middle). Apply relaxer to one half of your hair, process, rinse and shampoo with neutralizing shampoo. Then do the same process with the remainder of your hair. This will allow you to take your time with the application process without stressing out. Over and under processed patches in the hair will be minimized as well because you will be taking your time with the chemical process.

179. **ALWAYS neutralize your hair.** The relaxer will change the PH of your hair to 11-13 which is very basic.

The PH of your hair should be brought back down to 4.5 – 5. The neutralizing shampoo will drop the hair's PH because the hair cannot be left in a basic state. I have heard disaster stories of people relaxing their hair and not using a neutralizing shampoo after rinsing the relaxer from the hair. This will cause immediate hair loss within days. After relaxing, it is a great idea to allow the neutralizing shampoo to sit on the hair for at least 5 minutes (for 3 shampoos). This will insure that the PH levels are brought back to normal.

180. **Protecting your scalp.** Always base the scalp with some sort of oil before applying a relaxer. This will provide a light barrier and will slightly protect the scalp from burns and damage during the relaxing process.

181. **Protecting your hair ends.** Protecting your hair is crucial during the relaxing process. The goal is to protect the hair that has been previously relaxed. This can be done by applying oil or conditioner to your hair ends. This will prevent overlapping of the relaxer on previously relaxed hair.

182. **"Texturizing" can be a less damaging option.** If you want to slightly loosen your curl pattern without getting your hair very straight, texturizing may be for you. Texturizing will allow you to keep much of your curl pattern. It can easily be straightened as well so it will allow for much versatility. This can be done by applying the relaxer to your hair and letting it sit for just a few minutes before rinsing and following with a neutralizing shampoo. Your hair will not be super straight but your curl pattern will be slightly loosened.

183. **Permanent color and relaxed hair.** It is possible to color relaxed hair and not experience much breakage

but this should unquestionably be done by an expert. Based on my experience, going lighter is always more dangerous because a stronger developer needs to be used to lift the hair. This can be a disaster if not done professionally. It is best not to permanently color relaxed hair but if you must color your hair, be sure that you wait at least 2-3 weeks after your relaxer. Also, be sure that your hair is treated with a protein deep conditioning treatment prior to coloring the hair. This will strengthen the hair and prepare it for the chemical process. A healthier alternative is to use a rinse or semi-permanent color if you have a relaxer. Color rinses are safe because these colors only coat the hair strand and not penetrate. Rinses can be applied on the same day as your relaxer process. You cannot lighten your hair with a rinse.

184. **Protein treatments are a must before relaxing.** As briefly mentioned in the previous tip. It is a great idea to give yourself a protein treatment 1-2 weeks before your chemical process. Protein treatments will fill in the porous gaps in the hair. This will strengthen the hair shaft and prepare it for chemical processing.

185. **Boost those protein levels regularly!** Don't be afraid to boost your protein levels because if you are chemically treated, you will need the extra boost. Chemically treated hair tends to be a lot more porous and a bit more protein is needed to fill in the porous gaps. Schedule regular protein treatments in your hair care regimen to keep your hair healthy and strong. It will also help to prevent breakage by binding to the weakened areas and strengthening the hair.

LOCS

Locs are becoming more and more mainstream these days. As a loc wearer myself, I have noticed this first hand. Many people loc their hair for numerous reasons including spiritual / religious, low maintenance, life lessons and because they just love the look of locs. The ways in which locs are nurtured differ. There is not one strict method to cultivate and maintain locs. There are many ways to care for locs because they are very organic and develop on their own. If you are a new loc wearer on an experienced one, you will definitely benefit from the below hair tips that will keep your locs healthy and strong.

186. **Starting locs**. How you start your locs really depend on your lifestyle and the type of look that you are trying to achieve. There are many methods of starting locs and they all have pros and cons.
Free form- Just leaving the hair alone and letting your locs develop on their own. There is very little (if any) manipulation done to the hair. No twisting. You are just letting the hair do what it wants to do. The hair develops its own form of ever-changing art. Many celebrities have rocked free form locs including Lenny Kravitz, The Weeknd and Basquiat.
Comb coils- The hair is coiled with a comb in small sections. This will give the person a very neat and uniform cylindrical loc. The hair takes longer to loc this way. Coils give a very neat look as the hair locs.
Interlocking – The hair is sectioned off and interlocked with a crochet needle going in north / south / east / west directions. This way of starting locs is great for

those with active lifestyles because they will not unravel and you can wash them as often as you like. Interlocked locs will develop into a tighter/ thinner / more compact loc with a bit more shrinkage.

Braidlocs- Braiding the hair and letting the braid eventually form into a loc as time passes. This technique will give you a thinner loc as well. It is similar to interlocking technique because it will not unravel easily like comb coils. The braid pattern can remain in the loc for quite a long time. With some hair types, the braid pattern is permanent and some individuals may or may not like this look.

Crochet technique- This technique is also known as "instant dreadlocks". This is how I started my locs. It is usually done on very soft or straighter hair textures but it can be done on any hair type. This will allow for the hair to loc quickly. This technique involves slightly back combing the hair and using a very small crochet needle to mat the hair. The crochet needle is used to weave the hair within itself by using a back and forth motion to form a loc. This technique is called "instant dreadlocks" because it will give the look of a mature loc right away.

Sisterlocks- This type of locking procedure utilizes a uniform locking grid with the help of a specialized sisterlocking tool. This look results in very small beautiful locks.

As you can see, there are many ways to start locs. The choice is yours.

187. **Water is your friend.** I have heard some people say that locs shouldn't be washed for 2-3 months after the install and to only use which hazel on the scalp. This is terrible advice! This can cause scalp infections

and buildup within the loc. Whether your locs are young or mature, water is your buddy. Water is the ultimate form of moisture and hydration so it is a great idea to spritz your hair will water daily or even wet it in the shower every few days if you wish. Water will actually aid in the loc'ing process so don't be afraid to get your new locs wet. If your starter locs are in comb coils, just cover with a stocking cap before wetting the hair.

188. **Experiencing loc buildup?** Deep cleanse as needed to remove buildup from the hair and scalp. Every so often, it is a great idea to remove possible loc buildup by deep cleaning your locs with a baking soda / apple cider vinegar mix. The baking soda and vinegar will bond with the buildup that may be imbedded in the loc and break it down. The hair can be soaked in a baking soda / acv rinse bath for 10-15 minutes then rinsed. The key is to prevent loc buildup before it starts by using water soluble products to care for your locs. I.e. Hydratherma Naturals products. (Shameless plug ☺) You can prevent any excess build up in the first place by cleansing weekly with a great cleansing shampoo. Product recommendations: Hydratherma Naturals Moisture Boosting Shampoo.

189. **Combat dryness.** Many people with locs suffer from dryness especially if the locs are color treated. I have seen dry locs completely break off on the ends and sometimes at the root area. Moisturizing with a water based moisturizer is very important because it will not leave buildup within the loc. Using oils on the hair is great but oil alone will not moisturize the hair. Product recommendation: Hydratherma Naturals Daily Moisturizing Growth Lotion after each shampoo.

190. **Don't over moisturize locs.** This is applicable to newbies. Over moisturizing the hair will cause the hair to be too soft and will slow the loc'ing process. It will also attract more lint which is what you absolutely don't want. Moisturizing with your water based moisturizer weekly after shampooing the hair should suffice.

191. **Avoid styles that cause too much tension around the hair line.** Many loc updos can cause irreversible hair loss if worn for long periods of time. I have seen many loc styles posted online and I just cringe because the style looks to be pulling the follicles directly out of the scalp. I have also seen many loc wearers with very thin hairlines resulting from wearing these types of styles. The follicles along the hair line are the most fragile and must be treated with care. I'm shocked that some stylist purposefully style the hair so tightly knowing that their client's hairline is already thinning. If you are wearing a style that is adding too much tension to the hairline-> 1) Tell your stylist to adjust the look so less tension results. 2) Be sure to massage your edges with a moisturizer or hair oil to prevent damage. 3) Don't wear the loc style for more than a few days. As mentioned previously in the braiding section......Take charge. If you feel that your hair style is uncomfortable, let your stylist know right away. Your hairstyle should not be painful.

192. **Deep condition as needed to prevent breakage.** Many disagree on whether or not individuals should deep condition locs. I believe that deep conditioning locs will strengthen them and prevent breakage and thinning. If your locs are color treated, this is particularly true because color treated hair needs

that extra TLC to prevent breakage. A great protein deep treatment (during your loc maintenance) will do the trick and keep your locs in tip top shape. Be sure to completely rinse the deep conditioner from your locs. Rinse very well.

193. **Don't "over condition" your locs.** Using a moisturizing deep conditioning treatment (as needed) is absolutely fine. It will add much needed moisture to your locs. As mentioned in the previous tip, I actually recommend it. The problem comes with over conditioning locs. This will cause the locs to become too soft. It may even cause unraveling at the end of the loc. What is "too much" you may ask? It will vary from person to person. Try deep conditioning with a moisturizing deep treatment once a month and see how your hair does. Increase and decrease the frequency based on your hair's needs.

194. **Dilute your shampoos and deep conditioners if necessary.** If you feel as though your deep conditioner or shampoo is too heavy for your locs but it has the attributes that you really love, don't throw it out. Dilute it a bit with water and then apply. You can even use an applicator bottle to make the application process easier.

195. **Locs and moisture / protein balance.** The same premise holds true for locs. Over moisturizing can cause your locs to become too soft and the use of too much protein can cause your locs to become hard. Balanced hair will break less and will be become healthier over time. You can alternate your protein and moisture deep treatment every 4-8 weeks to encourage moisture / protein balance. This will prevent the hair from getting too soft or too hard which leads to breakage.

196. **Stay away from waxes, grease, and heavy pomades.** I remember when I was in cosmetology school in the 1990's and beeswax was the "go to" product to start locs with. Loc gels and foams were not popular products to start locs with back then. Now we know that waxes and products that contain mineral oil and petrolatum will cause MAJOR buildup which is extremely difficult to remove from locs. I have even heard of individuals using sticky HONEY to start locs! Ewwwwww……Choose water based products for retwists and general grooming. Light gels and foams work much better.
Product recommendation- The water based Hydratherma Naturals Botanica Defining Gel or the Foaming Sea Silk Curly Styler for loc maintenance.
197. **Retwist methods.** If you want your retwist to last longer, retwist on clean hair that is wet or slightly damp. This method will last a lot longer when compared to retwisting dry hair.
198. **Don't retwist or interlock too frequently.** This can cause loc thinning, thinning along the hairline, and loc breakage. Try to retwisting monthly (or slightly longer if possible) and be sure to keep your new growth well moisturized and healthy.
199. **Be sure that your locs are absolutely dry before retiring to bed.** Air drying is great but it is better to sit under a hood dryer to make sure that your locs are completely dry before going to bed. If you want to air dry, try cleansing earlier in the day to give your locs an ample amount of time to dry. Going to sleep with wet locs can cause the hair and scalp to be a haven for mold growth. This can cause your locs to smell like

mildew in the morning. This is something that you absolutely don't want.

200. **Avoid very tight interlocking.** If you like to maintain your locs with interlocking, be sure that it is not done too often and not done very tight. This will cause extreme stress to the hair follicles, permanent hair loss and breakage. How often you interlock will definitely depend on the look that you are going for and the rate of your hair growth. Some people interlock every month and some individuals go longer. Just make sure that your follicles are not strained when you interlock.

201. **Avoiding lint.** Huuummmm......This lint issue will be an ongoing one if you are a loc wearer. It is something that you constantly have to be conscious of so that it will not get out of control. Prevention is the key because once the lint is embedded in the loc, it will be very difficult to remove without weakening the actual loc. There are many super easy ways to prevent "the lint issue" but the most important thing to do is to protect your hair. Cover your hair at night and during the day if you are in dusty areas or if you are doing house work. Use a satin or silk pillowcase and dry your hair with a tee shirt or micro fiber towel that matches your hair color. If your locs are mature, try brushing your locs daily to help to remove surface lint.

202. **Existing lint.** If you are already suffering from lint pieces that are deeply embedded in your loc, I don't suggest that you dig into the loc with needles and such to remove the lint pieces. This will only damage your loc and cause it to unravel. It will also cause thinning in the area. I would rather you preserve your loc and cover

the small area affected by the lint. You can do this with the help of a temporary color rinse, black tea rinse or by color treating your hair with a semi-demi- or permanent hair color. I have heard of individuals even using permanent markers to color the lint the same color as their hair. Not sure about the marker but it is nice to know that you have options.

203. **Still insist on pulling out lint with a tweezer or needle????** This is a tricky one. As mentioned previously, this method to remove lint can be damaging to the loc so be very careful before you bring out those tweezers. If you do choose this method, try it on wet or damp hair. Water will expand the loc and make the lint a bit easier to remove.

204. **Know that deep cleansing your locs will not remove lint embedded in the loc.** I have read online about people attempting to remove lint with the help of deep cleansing treatments such as apple cider vinegar / baking soda washes. There is no cleaning solution that will remove lint that is deeply embedded within the loc. Deep cleansing will do an excellent job with removing product buildup but the lint will remain.

205. **Protective style.** When you hear the words "Protective Style", you automatically think of styles for loose natural hair. Protective styling is not just for loose naturals. Using protective styles on your locs will protect your hair from dusty environments and will help prevent the accumulation of lint and dirt in your locs. Wearing buns, braids and twist are cute and fun protective styles to wear.

206. **Colored locs.** I absolutely love the look of colored locs. Bright reds, blondes, shiny black and

purple shades are my absolute favorites. The funkier, the better! Coloring locs can be a bit tricky. If done incorrectly, it can lead to damage. Color damage can lead to breakage and loc thinning which is something that you definitely want to stay far away from. I definitely suggest that color treating your locs be done by a licensed professional who is experienced in coloring loc'd hair. This is especially true if you are lightening your locs because lightened hair is more prone to damage. If you do decide to take the plunge and color your own locs, be sure not to make the mistake of squeezing the color into the loc. Just lightly apply the color to the outside and pat through. Squeezing the color into the loc may make the color extremely difficult to remove which can cause loc damage and thinning. Also…. be sure to remove all of the color by rinsing extremely well and shampooing the hair after your color treatment. You want to be sure that all of the chemical is removed. You do not want to leave any of the color treatment in your loc. This will result in serious loc damage.

207. **Don't over use oils.** Being too heavy handed with oils will cause your hair to attract lint and dust. Typically, it is not necessary to apply oil on a daily basis. Oils are great to use but only use as needed. There is not an oil regimen that suits everyone. Just listen to your hair and it will tell you what it needs.

208. **Don't be afraid to use protein treatments on your locs.** This is certainly true if your locs are color treated. This will help minimize breakage. Many are under the assumption that loc'd hair will not break. This is far from the truth. Loc'd hair can definitely experience

breakage. This will typically occur at the hair root / new growth area. Loc wearers can also experience breakage at the end of the loc. Protein treatments will help to strengthen the hair and prevent this type of breakage. Product recommendation: Hydratherma Naturals Amino Plus Protein Deep Conditioning Treatment.

209.   **Avoid the "hand in hair syndrome".** Sometimes loc wearers can constantly play in their hair. I must admit that I am guilty of this at times. I definitely understand how tempting it can be. There is something about feeling all of those coils and kinks forming into ever-changing artwork on your head. As tempting as it may be, try to limit twisting and twirling your locs on a daily basis because it can absolutely lead to breakage and weak areas along the loc.

TRANSITIONING OUT OF THE RELAXER

Have you decided to say no to the relaxer? Many people stop relaxing their hair for countless reasons. It could be due to hair damage, scalp damage, hair loss or cultural / personal reasons. I personally decided to "go natural" because I really missed my feeling my natural curl pattern that I had come to love so much. I felt more comfortable wearing my hair natural as well. Transitioning out of the relaxer can be a very challenging time. Breakage at the line of demarcation is one major challenge. Styling options can also be slightly difficult due to managing two different hair textures. Mentally adjusting to your new natural texture can be a trial as well because many individuals are going natural for the first time and have absolutely no experience with maintaining their hair in its 100% natural state. Many of our transitioning customers stated to me that they haven't even seen their natural hair since they were small children. Transitioning out of the relaxer can be a difficult challenge but below are some tips that will make your life a lot easier as you go through the process.

210. **Know that a relaxer cannot be stripped from your hair.** I often receive emails from customers asking if they could use some sort of solution to strip the relaxer out of the hair. The truthful answer is no. I have heard many false tales of people stripping the relaxer out of their hair with eggs or peanut butter concoctions. These rumors are absolutely false. The relaxed ends are permanently straightened because the bonds in the hair have been permanently changed. The relaxed hair has

to be cut out all at once AKA big chop grown out over time.

211. **Big chop or no???** If you desire to go natural, there are 2 ways to do it. One way is to do the "big chop". This is the adventurous route which involves letting your relaxer grow out for a few months and then cutting all of your relaxed hair off. This usually results in a cute and sassy look called the TWA- Teenie Weenie Afro. This is the road that I went on when I first went natural. I went without a relaxer for about 5 months and then I cut off my relaxed ends. The feeling that I felt after cutting my hair was indescribable. I felt totally liberated and free. For those who did the big chop in the past…….you absolutely know the feeling. I felt so excited about my new natural hair journey. I was so thrilled about all of the fun that I was going to experience with my hair as it transitioned from super short to long.

212. **The long transition.** Some people freak out at the thought of doing the big chop. I know that it horrifies many. If the big chop is not for you, don't fret. There is another alternative. You can grow your hair out over longer periods of time and slowly snip off the relaxed ends every few months. If you go this route, you can hold on to your length. This is called the long transition. It is a great option for those who don't like the look of short hair. If you are one to live on the wild side, go for the big chop. It's much more fun!

213. **Be extremely gentle with your hair as you transition.** The hair is most prone to breakage during the transitioning phase because the hair is very weak at the line of demarcation. As mentioned previously, the

line of demarcation is the area along the strand where the relaxed hair ends and the natural hair begins. This is a very fragile area along the hair strand. The relaxed hair will tend to pop off easily because the natural hair is much more resilient. For this reason, it is very important to keep you hair well moisturized and handled with care during this time.

214. **Breakage is inevitable during the transition process.** You cannot transition out of your relaxer without experiencing some form of breakage. Just realize that some breakage will occur during the transitioning process. The key is to minimize breakage. Breakage can be reduced by following healthy hair care practices but it cannot be completely eliminated. This is because the chemically processed hair is weaker than your natural hair. If you see a bit more hair in the comb, don't be too alarmed. It is all a part of the process.

215. **Protein Treatments are top priority as you transition.** Schedule regular protein treatments in your hair care regimen. The protein will bind to the weakened areas along the line of demarcation and will strengthen the hair. Reinforcing the weakened areas will help to minimize some of the breakage that you will experience as you transition. Don't opt for very heavy protein treatments because it will leave the hair too hard which will lead to more breakage. Go for for a lighter protein treatment that will add light proteins to the hair a little at a time.
Product recommendation: Hydratherma Naturals Amino Plus Protein Deep Conditioning Treatment

216. **New Growth Care.** Keep your new growth very soft and well moisturized as you transition. Moisturizing

your new growth daily is crucial to prevent breakage at the line of demarcation. Keeping the hair soft and moisturized will also make your new growth easier to manipulate which will prevent breakage. If your new growth is very dry and brittle, extreme breakage and damage will definitely occur.

Transitioning can be a serious "mental adjustment" and you do not need any added stress in the form of extreme breakage during this sensitive time. Hair loss at this time can be very traumatizing so just be sure to moisturize your new growth and avoid any extra anguish. Product Recommendations- Hydratherma Naturals Follicle Mist and Daily Moisturizing Growth Lotion

217. **Try braids!** Braids can be great protective styles if done properly. If you are not interested in doing the big chop or the long transition, wearing braids is a great style to rock as you grow your hair out. While wearing braids you can let your hair "rest" for a while as it grows. Once your hair becomes a comfortable length for you, you can wear your own hair with confidence. I do not recommend keeping braids in for longer than 5 weeks without giving your hair a breather for a few weeks. Keeping your hair braided for 4-5 weeks would be most advantageous to prevent breakage.

218. **Have your favorite fly "go to" style.** Dealing with 2 different textures can be a challenge so you always want to have that "go to" hair style that you can depend on when times get rough. With that "go to style" in your pocket, your hair will always look good in case you are in a rush or if the weather isn't great. Great options are limitless and include creative buns,

braided styles, large flat twist styles or a curly puff. These types of "go to" styles also do not require much combing and manipulation of the hair. Low manipulation is very important while transitioning so that breakage will be minimized.

219. **Straightening your new growth as you transition.** I have seen many transitioners make this tragic mistake so many times. If you would like to wear the straight look as you transition, be very careful to avoid heat damage. Many transitioners tend to overuse heat in an attempt to match their natural new growth with their relaxed ends. In many cases, the new growth is being blasted with high heat on a regular basis. Once the relaxer has grown out, the natural hair is lifeless and harmed beyond repair. Many people will have to cut their hair off and begin their natural hair journey again. This experience can be heartbreaking. To avoid this, try roller sets as you transition while blowing out the roots only (with medium heat). If you have to use direct heat, I would suggest using ceramic or tourmaline styling tools because they are far less damaging. Try not to use heat more than once a week on clean hair only.

220. **Curly styles reign while transitioning!** This is the TRUTH! If you are transitioning and wear straight styles all of the time, the humidity will cause a flawless hairstyle to look like a nightmare. Working with 2 different textures is very difficult if you wear straight looks frequently as you transition. It can also be very damaging (see previous tip). Have fun with styles that will last through the humidity. Try bantu knot sets, braid outs, rod sets, straw sets and twist outs. These types of styles require less manipulation. Just finger comb in the

morning and you are out of the door. With styles like these, you can go the gym and still keep your cute curly style! You also don't have to worry so much about sweating out your roots.

221. **As you transition, manipulate you hair very little**. I would suggest combing your hair on wash days only and not combing while it is in its dry state. This will cut down on the breakage that you may experience to a great extent. If you are wearing curly styles just finger comb in the morning. If you are wearing your hair straight, comb with a wide tooth comb (if necessary) and try to manipulate your hair very little.

222. **Keep a great hair regime**. Sticking with a consistent routine is crucial as you transition out of your relaxer. Washing and treating your hair weekly with a deep conditioning treatment remains very important during the transitioning phase. Be sure to maintain a healthy protein / moisture balance in your hair as well. Your hair is in its most fragile state during your transitioning months and keeping the hair balanced will prevent some of the breakage that you may experience.

223. **Have patience**. Transitioning will not happen overnight. It takes lots of fortitude and perseverance so just hang in there! As your hair grows out, slowly trim off the relaxed ends and soon all of the relaxed ends will be gone. If your hair grows 1/2 inch per month, you can expect about 6 inches in 1 year. If you can't stand to wait that long, you can always do the big chop!

224. **Be careful with sew-in weaves.** Many people opt to wear sew-in weaves as they transition out of their relaxer because it can serve as a great protective style. It is an awesome alternative if done correctly. If

you decide to wear a straight textured sew-in weave, opt for a "full sew-in" with no hair left out. If you leave some of your hair out to blend with the straight commercial hair, you will have to use a lot of heat on your natural hair for the perfect blend. This can be extremely damaging to your natural hair that has been left out for blending. I have seen many transitioners (with partial weaves) experience damage to the hair left out due to using massive amounts of heat. Once the transitioning process is over, the natural hair that was left out would be completely straight and the rest of the hair would be kinky and curly. If you would like a more natural looking sew-in weave with some of your hair left out, opt for a curly weave so that your real hair will blend easier.

COLOR TREATED HAIR

Many of us like to shake things up a bit with some fun hair color. There is something about the spring and summer that makes you just wanna try a red or a honey blonde just for the fun of it. Coloring the hair can be risky at times because color treated hair tends to be very porous and dry. Hair that has been treated with color can break off easily if not taken care of properly. There are ways to keep your colored tresses as healthy as possible. Check out these hair care tips to prevent breakage.

225. **Seek a professional with color experience.** This is always the best option when it comes to coloring your hair. This is especially true if you desire to "go lighter". If you decide to color your hair yourself be aware that it can be complicated as well as extremely risky. Many people underestimate how damaging it can be to lighten the hair. When I was a young adult, I colored my hair with a high lift box color and all of my hair fell out in bunches around my hairline. It was devastating and I was deathly afraid to color my hair again for years after that horrible experience. If you are not sure and confident in this type of chemical processes, please seek a professional with color experience. It is better to be safe than sorry. Having healthy color treated hair is definitely worth the investment.

226. **For a "damage free" color change, try a temporary color rinse.** A rinse will only last for 1-2 shampoos but it will not damage your hair at all. It can last a bit longer on porous hair. It will only coat the hair strand because it is ammonia and peroxide free. It will

not penetrate the hair strand and because of this, you cannot lift the hair to lighter hues. You can go darker or add a hint of red with this option. I sometimes like to use rinses to add a rich shiny black to my hair without the commitment. Color rinses are very beneficial to the hair as well because it coats the hair strand but still allows moisture to enter. This coating protects the cuticle, buffers heat and gives the hair a nice shine. It may also prevent breakage. The disadvantage is that the color may "bleed". This can be a deal breaker for some because it can bleed on your clothing if you are caught in the rain. It can also bleed on your pillow cases and collars which can be a drag.

227. **For best results, be sure that your hair is clean when the hair color is applied.** Hair loaded with buildup will not absorb the hair color evenly. This can result in color variations and unpleasant light and dark spots. You can gently cleanse the hair and scalp 1-2 days before coloring your hair. Try not to scratch your scalp while cleansing the hair to avoid scalp irritation during the coloring process. Don't add heavy oils and moisturizers to your hair right before coloring. You want to begin with a clean slate so that the hair color will be absorbed evenly along the hair shaft.

228. **Want a little extra shine?** Try a clear rinse. If your natural hair color looks dull, you can try a clear color just to give your hair a boost of shine. There are many clear deposit only "colors" brands to choose from. These clear hair colors will add a nice gloss to your hair without adding any tint. These varieties of clear hair colors come in semi, demi and permanent colors. I would recommend the semi or demi color choices

because they are less harmful to the hair. Clear semi-permanent rinses have the same benefits as color rinses and will protect the cuticle as well.

229. **Colored hair needs that extra TLC in the form of protein.** I'm sure that you have seen many individuals with extremely damaged color treated hair. Color treated hair can break easily if it isn't taken care of properly. It also tends to be a lot more porous and needs a bit more protein to fill in the porous gaps. Once the porous gaps are filled with added protein, the hair will be strengthened and breakage will be prevented. When you see someone with beautiful and healthy color treated hair, you now know their secret……..Adding protein to their healthy hair regimen is key.

230. **Be careful …too much protein is not a good idea.** Now that we know all about color treated hair needing more protein, we should not go too crazy with the harsh protein treatments. I remember casually mentioning to an acquaintance about color treated hair needing additional protein. I later found out that she began to give her hair harsh protein treatments weekly. When I saw her a few months later, her color treated hair was thin and breaking. She began to tell me about what she was doing to her hair. I realized right away that she was experiencing protein overload. I explained to her that adding too much protein to her hair can cause severe damage (resulting in breakage). A great tip would be to skip the heavy treatments and use light protein treatments 2 x per month. This is a great way to increase her protein levels safely without experiencing protein overload and breakage. Your stylist will be able

to let you know if your protein levels are up to par. If you want to know for yourself, see the moisture / protein balance section of this book for tips and tricks. Product recommendation- Hydratherma Naturals Amino Protein Deep Conditioning Treatment.

231. **Moisturize / Moisturize / Moisturize-** I just can't express this enough. We all know that color treated hair is prone to dryness and breakage. This dryness can be extreme and can cause breakage / hair loss. Excessive dryness is typically associated with high lift colors. Blondes and light reds tend to cause more dryness and damage because most of these types of colors use ammonia and peroxide. In addition to adding protein (as mentioned in the previous tips), moisture needs to be added to your hair regimen to keep the hair balanced. As mentioned previously, color treated hair is very porous so keeping it balanced is vital.

232. **Prevent color treated hair from fading.** Everyone loves the way that their hair looks when they first get it colored. The reds and the honey blondes are the most vibrant! The down side is that the reds and the honey blondes fade the fastest. This will naturally occur as time passes but you can prevent accelerated color fading with the use sulfate free shampoos. The use of sls free cleansers will prevent excessive color fading because most sls free shampoos are color safe and less stripping.
Product recommendation –Hydratherma Naturals SLS FREE Moisture Plus Hair Cleanser.

233. **Beware of bleach.** Bleaching the hair can cause severe damage and immediate hair loss if done improperly. If growing out healthy and strong hair is

your ultimate goal, I would recommend that you completely avoid bleaching your hair. To be honest, is extremely challenging to grow healthy / long bleached hair. You will be fighting an uphill and unnecessary battle if you decide to go this route. If you don't have a desire to grow your hair long and you love the short look, bleach can be tolerated because you will not be trying to retain length. As the hair growths out, the damaged ends will get clipped off over time.

234. **Lightening your hair-** Lightening your hair should be done with extreme caution. If you would like to go a lot lighter, this cannot be done with a semi-permanent or a demi-permanent color. Lightening can only be done with a permanent color because ammonia and peroxide are both needed to lift and deposit the new hair color into your hair strands. Bleach is not necessary unless you are trying to achieve a very light blonde hair color. You can lift your hair to a light blonde with hair color which is a safer alternative compared to using bleach. As mentioned previously, going lighter requires that you do an extremely excellent job at keeping your hair balanced with moisture and protein to prevent breakage.

235. **Darkening your hair.** When it comes to coloring your hair, going darker is a much safer alternative. This is because there are many products that can be used to darken your hair without the use of ammonia or peroxide (very damaging components). Deposit only colors are the best alternative. Semi-permanent rinses are great but they only last for a few shampoos. It may last a bit longer if your hair is porous. My absolute favorite "deposit only" color type is the demi-

permanent color. I personally use this color myself and it fits my needs just perfectly. I use a black demi-permanent hair color every 3-4 months. It will last for about 24 shampoos without a retouch and it leaves my hair damage free. No need to go darker with an ammonia based permanent color at all. Team Demi! See more details on demi permanent colors at tip 239.

236. **Don't color your hair too often.** This is a common mistake that I see many people make. For optimal hair health, try not to apply permanent color more often than every 12 weeks. Also, only apply the permanent hair color to the new growth area and try not to overlap on previously colored hair. Overlapping hair color can be severely damaging. If you feel as though you have to color your hair more frequently, try rinses or semi-permanent color treatments in between touchups to keep your hair color fresh and vibrant.

237. **Try Henna powder to color your hair.** Although the coloring options are a bit limited with henna, it is a great option to give your hair a slightly reddish shade. It works well to cover grey as well. Be sure that the henna is 100% natural. Read the ingredients on the back of the package to be sure that no other chemicals have been added. The disadvantage is that henna takes a long time to apply, it can be very messy and must be left on for at least 2-8 hours. The benefits outweigh the disadvantages in my opinion. Henna is permanent, it does not fade and it gives the hair a very nice shine. It also has thickening properties. Henna can make your hair very dry so be sure to deep condition and moisturize your hair very well after the application. Another great thing about henna is that you can mix it

with other Indian powders to achieve other rich red, brown and black hues.

238. **Go jet black the 100% natural way!** Naturally color your hair jet black with Henna and Indigo powders. This is a natural way to permanently dye your hair black. It is a 2 step process. First, apply the henna powder and let it sit for 2-8 hours. The longer you let the henna process, the richer the red will be. The second step is to mix and apply the indigo power to your hair. The indigo only has to process for 2-4 hours. The down side is that it is very time consuming but the results are well worth it if you want to go the natural route. The shade of black will be long lasting and full of shine!

239. **Do you want a dark brown, black or dark red tone without the permanent commitment?** A demi permanent hair color may be the absolute best and safest choice for you. I briefly touched on the demi permanent option in a previous tip but it deserves its very own detailed section.

This is my absolute favorite type of color to use for "going darker" without the commitment or the damage. For ideal hair health and longer lasting color, demi permanent hair colors are the absolute safest. These types of colors are less damaging compared to permanent colors because they penetrate the hair strand very little. Demi permanent colors are ammonia free and contain small amounts of peroxide for color deposit to occur. You can use a 5 or 10 volume developer to deposit this type of color. You cannot go lighter with these types of colors because they only deposit the color in the strand and will not lift the hair.

These types of colors usually last for about 24 shampoos (with 10 volume developer) and 12 shampoos (with 5 volume developer). It can last a bit longer on hair that is has been previously chemically treated (relaxed or colored) or overly porous hair. I personally like to use the black demi color on my locs because I may want to change things up and go with a lighter color one day. If I decide to do that, it wouldn't be a problem at all because the demi color will be removed in 12-24 weeks. If my hair was permanently colored black and I wanted to go lighter, the black would be very difficult to lift and my hair would be prone to severe damage. Demi colors rock!

240. **Avoid scalp injury.** As with any chemical process avoid scratching your scalp prior to the coloring process (or any chemical process). This can cause burning. You cannot base the scalp for protection prior to coloring your hair as you would with a relaxer. It will interfere with the color process. To ensure an amazing color process from root to tip, be sure that your scalp is in great shape prior to coloring. If your scalp is damaged at all, postpone your color application until your scalp issue is resolved.

241. **Try color sprays or chalking for vibrant temporary colors!** This is a great way to experience a temporary color change that will last for a day or two before shampooing. There is a wide array of colors to choose from. Greens, blues, pinks, reds, purples etc. The choices are endless. The only disadvantage is that these colors bleed easily so be sure not to be caught in the rain. You'll be in big trouble.

242. **Change is good but…………….don't go overboard.** Changing your hair color often with permanent color may be exciting and fun but it can wreak havoc on your hair. There was a time in my teen years when I experimented a lot with color. I went from brown to blonde to red and back to a lighter blonde. The bad part is that these color changes occurred during one summer. What on earth was I thinking???? A few days after the last color process, my hair was coming out at the roots and I was completely bald on the right side of my head. Opting for semi perm, demi perm or temporary color sprays would have been better choices for me back then but as they say……. Hindsight is 20/20.

243. **Virgin hair colors.** If you are a DIYer (Do It Yourselfer), be sure to educate yourself on the virgin coloring process. If you opt to color your own hair and you are doing a "virgin" color, be sure to process your hair ends first (1 inch from the scalp to ends). Once the color is applied to the hair ends, proceed to apply the color to the root area. The color will process faster in the root area because of the natural heat that the scalp produces. This process will prevent a lighter color in the root area which we call "hot roots". It will also ensure an even color from root to tip.

244. **Prep your hair prior to your color application.** You definitely want your hair to be in optimal condition at the time of your color process. This can be done by adding light proteins to the hair shaft to fill in any porous gaps. Heavy proteins are not necessary. It is a great idea to give yourself a light protein treatment 1-2 weeks prior to color treating your hair. This will

strengthen your hair and prepare it for chemical processing. It will also even out the porosity in your hair so when color is applied, it will be absorbed by the hair strand evenly. This will avoid "hot spots" (aka uneven hair color) in porous areas.

Product recommendation – Hydratherma Naturals Amino Plus Protein Deep Conditioning Treatment

TRIMMING SPLIT ENDS

Trimming the hair is a very important aspect of any healthy hair journey. If you want to prevent breakage, trimming is absolutely necessary. This is very true for natural and chemically processed hair. How often you should trim and the method used will vary from person to person.

245. **The scissors are your best friend if you want to retain length.** Trimming your split ends will not make your hair grow any faster but it will prevent the split ends from working their way up the hair strands causing damage. If you decide to skip those trims, you will experience severe breakage because split ends will weaken the hair shaft. You will not experience length retention if this happens. Just remember that split ends will eventually break so prevent those splits before they start. If you trim regularly, you will retain inches as time goes by.

246. **Use super sharp shears only!** I suggest that you invest in a great pair of shears EXCLUSIVELY used for trimming your hair. Don't use the same scissors for household use. These special "hair shears" should be super sharp and only brought out for hair trimming. Using very sharp shears will give you a nice clean cut. Using dull scissors will cut each strand unevenly. This will cause the very ends of your hair strand to fray and will cause your hair ends to split even faster.

247. **If your ends are severely damaged, it is a great idea to cut off the damaged portion of your hair and just start from scratch.** Remember that split ends will break. If the split ends are not completely removed, the hair will continue to break so length and thickness will

not be obtained. Damaged hair cannot be made healthy again no matter what product you use or how much you deep condition. It is best to remove the damaged portion. Your cut doesn't have to be drastic but we suggest that you cut "just enough" so that the thin ends are removed.

248. **Don't be afraid to trim.** Realize that you will still retain length if your ends are clipped regularly. Some believe that clipping their ends does impede length retention. This is simply not true unless you are trimming too much or too often. Clipping off 1/8 to 1/4 inch every 2-3 months will still allow length to be retained. The average person experiences growth at the rate of 1/4- 1/2 inch per month.

249. **Prevent the "SEVERITY" of split ends.** You can't stop split ends from occurring but you can definitely prevent the "severity" of split ends. This can be done by preventing damage to the hair shaft before it starts. Using heat, blow dryers, chemical applications and even combing / brushing too frequently will cause split ends to occur more often. Handle your hair with a little TLC and you will notice a decrease in the occurrence of split ends. You will also notice that eventually your hair will start to thicken.

250. **Do you have chemically treated hair?** If so, you may need to trim a bit more often. If your hair is chemically processed in any way (color treated, relaxed, texlaxed etc.), clipping your hair every 8-10 weeks is typically enough. Chemically treated hair tends to need trimming more often because it is more porous. Porous hair has gaps along the hair strand and this contributes to split ends. If your hair is all natural and you do not

use heat appliances often, you can get by with trimming once or twice a year. Everyone's hair is a bit different but your hair will let you know what it needs.

251. **Trim Schedule.** There is not a "one size fits all" trim schedule that everyone must abide by. A trim schedule will vary from person to person depending on your hair type and hair care practices. The important thing is to prevent split ends before they start. Some can get by with trimming every 8 weeks and others can trim yearly without any problems. As mentioned previously, hair that is chemically processed needs to be trimmed more frequently. If you habitually use heat, you may have to trim more often as well. You can choose the best trim schedule by starting with a fresh trim and seeing how long it takes for your ends to slightly start splitting. This time period is different for everyone but just keep a close eye on your hair ends as the weeks go by. Based on that time period, you can schedule out your trims as needed.

252. **Kinky textures and split ends.** It can be very common for those with kinky hair textures to not trim as often as necessary. I was guilty of this mistake early into my natural hair journey. I went over a year once without trimming. I typically wore my hair in really curly afros and seeing frizz wasn't unusual. When I decided to straighten my hair, I was really able to visualize the negative effects of not trimming. My ends were splitting severely and my hair was very uneven. At that moment, I decided not to go that long without a trim again. If your hair is naturally curly and/or kinky, it can sometimes be easy to ignore split ends because they may not be easily visible or felt. Damaged ends may

not be caught early enough if they are not obviously seen. This can result in an unfortunate hair setback.

253. **Use the twist and clip technique.** This is the easiest way to clip your ends and works best on kinky or curly hair textures. Section the lair in 1 cubic inch section. Two strand twist the section and clip ¼ - ½ inch from the end of the twist. This technique will not give you a precision trim but it works like a charm and does the job!

254. **Search and destroy method.** Not for the weak at heart! This technique is only for the dedicated because it can take many hours! This technique entails sectioning the hair and searching each section for split ends ………..one strand at a time. If you use this method, you will only clip the ends that need trimming and leaving the rest. This is very time consuming but some swear by it for length retention. If you have at least 2-4 hours to spare, give it a go and see how it works for you.

255. **Realize that split ends cannot be mended.** Once the hair strand splits, it cannot be repaired and it will continue to split up the hair shaft until the strand breaks. There is not a miracle product that will repair split ends. It just doesn't exist. There are products that will help hold the cuticle together and prevent the hair from splitting as fast. These products contain ceramides which are lipid molecules. These lipid molecules act as a glue to hold the cuticle layer in place. It makes the cuticle stronger and prolongs the length of time before splitting occurs. Ceramides will not permanently repair split ends.

Product rich in ceramides include our product

recommendations: Hydratherma Naturals Protein Balance Leave In Conditioner, Daily Moisturizing Growth Lotion and the Hair Growth Oil.

256. **Trichoclasis.** Split hairs along the hair shaft. Trichoclasis occurs when the hair strand splits midway along the hair shaft. The end of the hair strand may or may not be intact. Once this occurs, the strand will typically break at the split site. Prevention is key. Trichoclasis is typically caused by excessive hair damage and bad hair care practices. Decreasing the use of heat and chemicals will help prevent Trichoclasis.

HAIR LOSS

Hair loss is a very serious issue among women and men. The loss of hair can be especially devastating to women and can cause serious self-esteem issues. Hair loss may result from many different causes including hereditary issues, medications/ health issues, nutritional deficiencies, stress and even a lack of sleep. Here are a few of the major causes of hair loss and some possible remedies. If you notice changes in your hair suddenly or over time, consult your health care professional to see if there is an internal cause.

257. **Menopause and hair loss.** Going through the "Change of Life" can definitely cause hair loss among many women. Menopause can also affect the rate of hair growth a woman experiences. Hair loss related to menopause typically results from an imbalance of hormones. If you are experiencing menopause symptoms along with hair loss or slow growth, seek your medical professional. They can help you to balance your hormones by initiating some type of hormone replacement therapy. Once your hormones are balanced, your hair loss issues should slowly resolve as time passes.

258. **Medication and hair loss.** Be mindful of your medication's side effects. Some medications can have negative effects on the hair such as hair thinning and slow growth. Blood pressure medications, birth control pills, thyroid medications and many other meds have "hair loss" listed as common side effects. If you have noticed changes in your hair after taking a certain

medication, consult your health care professional to see if your prescription medication can be the cause.

259. **Heavy alcohol consumption and hair loss.** Alcohol affects the liver's metabolic processes. If the liver is even slightly distressed, it can affect how your body metabolizes vitamins and minerals essential for hair growth and general health. If our body is unable to process vitamins and minerals properly, just imagine the negative affect that this can have on your hair and overall health.

260. **Improper digestion and hair loss / slow growth.** Proper digestion is an absolute must. Just think....if your body is unable to properly digest the food that you eat, the nutrients will not be disseminated properly to your cells. This will result in nutritional deficiencies. If you are suffering from any type of digestive issues, it is imperative to heal your gut. It is very important that your body's digestive system is healthy so that you will be able to break down your food properly and absorb the proper nutrients necessary for healthy hair growth and general health. One way to do this is by following an anti-inflammatory diet. A traditional Paleo or Paleo Vegetarian diet can help reduce gastrointestinal inflammation and will help your gut to heal. I have been eating this way for the last 5 years and digestive problems are a thing of the past for me. The diet also helped me to lose 30 lbs. and get off of all of my medications. That was an added plus ☺ Tip- Digestive enzyme supplements will help you to break down your food properly so that you will be better able to absorb the nutrients that your body

needs. The l-glutamine amino acid and probiotics will also help to heal your gut.

261. **Pregnancy and hair loss.** Hormonal changes during pregnancy and the physical stressors that occur during birth can cause hair loss. The hair loss is typically seen after the baby has been born. During the pregnancy the hair grows very fast and flourishes. After the birth, the hair may start to shed. If you are experiencing hair loss, what should you do? Unless the shedding is extremely excessive, try not to worry too much. It is normal. With a healthy diet, your hormonal levels will normalize and your hair will naturally grow back and thicken.

262. **Birth control pills / female hormonal issues and hair loss.** Starting, stopping or changing hormonal birth control methods can cause telogen effluvium (temporary thinning of hair) and/ or slow growth. Many women notice changes in their hair after starting or changing their birth control methods. If you are experiencing any type of hormonal issues that may be affecting your hair, speak with your medical provider. He or she may change you birth control method and this may resolve your hair issues.

263. **Hereditary -Female pattern hair loss.** This is called androgenic or androgenetic alopecia. It is the female version of male pattern baldness. This typically runs in families. If many of the ladies in your family experience hair loss and thinning after a certain age, there is a higher chance that you may as well. Male pattern baldness typically presents with a receding hairline. With androgenetic alopecia, a generalized

thinning may occur. With this type of hair loss, topical treatments may not help because of the genetic factor. Unfortunately, there is not much that can be done about this type of thinning because it is hereditary. Hair replacement procedures may be an option for some individuals dealing with female pattern hair loss.

264. **Anemia and hair loss.** Almost one in 10 women aged 20 through 49 suffer from anemia due to an iron deficiency. Many African American women are affected because black women suffer from fibroids at a higher rate. Heavy bleeding related to fibroids can easily lead to anemia. Your health care provider will be able to run blood work to see if anemia is evident. Typically, this cause of hair loss is a simple issue to fix. An iron supplement should correct the problem and immediately stop the hair loss. If your anemia is related to fibroids, I suggest that you consult your physician to discuss your fibroid treatment options. Treating the fibroids will resolve the anemia if heavy menstrual bleeding is the cause of your anemia.

265. **Thyroid issues and hair loss.** An underactive thyroid gland aka hypothyroidism can unquestionably cause hair loss and thinning. The thyroid gland produces hormones that are needed for metabolism. When your body is not producing enough thyroid hormones, hair loss and slow growth can be evident. Weight gain can also be evident as slower metabolic processes present. Your medical provider can easily draw bloodwork to test your thyroid levels. Synthetic thyroid medication will be helpful in getting your metabolism back on track and will help with the hair loss issue as well.

266. **Feed your body healthy oils and stay away from unhealthy oils / trans fats.** Consume healthy oils such as flaxseed oil, fish oil (omega 3 fatty acids), olive oil, coconut oil and oil from avocados. These oils will increase sebum production which will lead to a healthy / moisturized scalp. Consuming these healthy oils may also aid in decreasing dandruff with some individuals. Increasing your intake of healthy oils will also result in soft, shiny and healthy hair.

267. **Extreme diets and hair loss.** There are so many extreme diets out there. Some of the titles are quite funny. Here are a few. The cabbage diet, the cookie diet and the lemon juice diet are some popular extreme ones. These diets will eventually cause nutritional deficiencies and the first place that you will notice a change is in your hair, skin and nails. This will serve as a warning that you are not receiving your proper nutrients. You will notice hair loss and excessive shedding because of the nutritional deficits that these diets present. I advise that you stay away from fad diets and make healthy eating a part of your daily lifestyle.

268. **Emotional stress and hair loss.** Try to stay as "stress free" as possible. I know that this is easier said than done but try not to live a life full of pressure, anxiety and tension. This will definitely affect your hair in a negative way. Stress can trigger hormones that can slow growth by disrupting the growth phase of the hair growth cycle. Stress and worry can also cause inflammation, diffuse hair loss and can trigger the onset of hereditary hair loss (or accelerate its progression). Try to identify what your stressors are and find ways to possibly remove them from your life. If the stressors

cannot be eliminated, find ways to cope with them. To deal with daily stress try yoga, meditation and prayer to calm your nerves. These coping practices must be done on a regular basis to see results.

269. **Physical stress and hair loss.** Any type of physical trauma can cause temporary hair loss. This may include things such as surgery, pain or an acute or chronic illness. These physical stressors can trigger "telogen effluvium" which is a type of temporary hair loss. It is caused by a prolonged shedding cycle due to physical stress. Once these physical stressors are resolved, the excessive hair loss should stop.

270. **Rapid weight loss and extreme dieting.** Dramatic / sudden weight loss can certainly trigger hair loss. This is because sudden weight loss can cause stress to the body. There may also be vitamin and mineral deficiencies evident with extreme weight loss. When I was working as a Registered Nurse, I took care of bariatric patients undergoing gastric bypass surgery. These patients typically experience fast weight loss. With this surgery, the size of the stomach is decreased dramatically and after the surgery, the patient will only be able to take in extremely small amounts of food at one time. Sometimes the patients would come back to visit us after the drastic weight loss. I noticed that hair thinning was evident with most of the patients and this was most likely related to some sort of nutritional deficiency. As time passed, their hair thickened as the deficiency resolved. Slow and steady weight loss, a healthy diet loaded with foods containing vitamins / minerals (no junk food) and a high quality multivitamin will help to replace missing nutrients.

271. **Lack of sleep and hair loss.** Sleep does the body good. Many people underestimate how important sleep is. About 8-9 hours of sleep a night is adequate. Physical / mental stress and lack of sleep go hand in hand. Sleep deprivation is a form of stress and stress is something that you definitely want to minimize in your life. Emotional stress is one of the most commonly reported causes of sleep deprivation and sleep deprivation can cause emotional stress with irritability. As you can see, this can turn into a never ending cycle. A lack of sleep is not good for hair growth and bad for overall general health. Be sure to get your rest.

272. **Cigarettes (or hookah) and hair loss.** Did you know that 1 hour of smoking hookah is equivalent to 100 cigarettes??!! Heyyyyyyyy....... I'm not trying to stop anyone from having a little fun but the regular use of hookah (or cigarettes) is a surefire way to stunt hair growth and cause diffuse hair loss. Both hookah and cigarettes will slow hair growth drastically because they decrease circulation and cause the blood vessels to constrict. This can be devastating to all organs in the body. It affects hair growth by decreasing circulation to the hair follicle. This will cause less nutrients and oxygen to reach the hair root resulting in much slower hair growth and hair loss.

HEALTH & NUTRITION

Healthy hair starts from within. To ensure that your hair grows healthy and strong, you definitely need to feed your body healthy vitamins and nutrients. Here are some nutritional tips that will encourage healthy hair growth.

273. **Hair Vitamin Supplementation.** It is always better to receive your vitamins and nutrients from healthy food sources. With the typical diet, many desirable nutrients may still be missing. If you feel as though your diet may be lacking in some nutrients, I suggest that you supplement your diet with a high quality hair vitamin that supports healthy hair growth. By doing this, you will be able to provide your body with all of the nutrients that it needs for healthy hair and general health.
Product recommendation- Hydratherma Naturals Hair Growth Plus Vitamin with Biotin, MSM, Silica, Keratin, Hyalauronic acid, collagen and many other herbs extracts and vitamins to support healthy hair, skin and nails.

274. **Give MSM a try.** While taking supplements, be sure that your hair growth supplement contains MSM. MSM is an organosulfur compound that occurs naturally in plants. MSM is believed to extend the growth phase of the hair growth cycle. This can possibly speed up your hair growth process. If you are allergic to sulfur be sure to consult your health care professional before taking MSM or any supplement containing it.

275. **Water Water Water!** As I mentioned in a previous tip, water is the ultimate form of moisture in

our bodies so it is extremely important that we drink plenty of it. At least 8 glasses a day will properly keep you hydrated. Fruit juices and sodas are not the best options to hydrate the body because they are loaded with sugar which can cause inflammation. Inflammation can actually impede healthy hair growth. If you are not a water drinker, try infusing it with fruit. Adding lemons, strawberries and even cucumbers to your water will add vitamins and enhance the flavor as well.

276. **Eat a protein rich diet.** Hair consists of keratin which is a protein made of amino acids. Your body must produce or ingest these amino acids in order to grow healthy hair. Diets that are extremely low in amino acid proteins will result in hair that is weak and fragile. High protein sources include eggs, dairy and meat. You can also get your protein from non-animal sources. See next tip.

277. **Vegetarianism and protein intake.** If you love eating plant based, you can still ingest healthy levels of protein. You can incorporate protein shakes or protein bars into your diet to boost your protein levels. Healthy proteins are also available in many veggies including broccoli as well as legumes and brown rice. With a little research and meal planning, ingesting adequate amounts of plant based protein is not necessarily a difficult job.

278. **A lack of protein can be problematic when it comes to healthy hair growth.** If you are not getting enough protein in your diet, hair growth will be stunted because your body will naturally ration the protein and use it for other (more important) life sustaining metabolic activities. Your body will try to hold on to the

protein and the hair will be the last recipient of the distributed protein. Hair loss may begin to occur within two to three months after your protein intake has dropped significantly.

279.   **Vitamins B7, C and E Rock!** Eat a diet high in vitamin B7 (encourages growth and helps to reduce hair loss), Vitamin C (helps to grow and strengthen hair) & Vitamin E (encourages sebum production for a healthy scalp). Stock up on your fruits, veggies, nuts and healthy meats (or other high protein sources) to get these vitamins naturally. If you decide to use supplements, just be sure that you are not taking more than the recommended daily allowance.

280.   **Vitamin A is great for your hair but too much vitamin A may be problematic.** When taking supplements, remember that more doesn't always mean better. This is especially true for the fat soluble vitamins A,D,E and K. Fat soluble vitamins are stored in the body for longer periods of time and can pose a greater risk for toxicity when consumed in excess. Taking too much Vitamin A may contribute to hair loss according to the American Academy of Dermatology. Vitamin A is fat soluble and your body will store any excess that you take in. This can result in toxicity resulting in hair loss. Make sure that you are not taking more than the recommended daily allowance. The Daily Value for vitamin A is 5,000 International Units (IU) per day for adults.

EXERCISE AND HAIR GROWTH

Exercise is very important when it comes to promoting hair growth and preventing hair loss. Many people overlook the correlation between exercise and healthy hair growth. In this section, I will discuss how important this correlation really is. I will also discuss how to manage our hair while exercising so that we won't let our hairstyles prevent us from being active.

281. **Exercise and hair growth.** Are you hitting the gym to lose weight or just to get a lot healthier? Getting fit is awesome but the increase in your hair growth rate is a wonderful added benefit. Many people who exercise on a regular basis may experience faster hair growth. I noticed this right away when I began exercising. My hair started growing like weeds. This happens because exercising increases blood flow to the scalp and hair follicles. The added blood flow provides much needed nutrients and oxygen to the hair root causing faster hair growth.

282. **Hairstyles and Exercising.** So you go to the hair salon and get that super cute silk press and Lord knows that you don't wanna sweat it out! You decide to take a few weeks off from your workouts so that you can be sure to get your money's worth. Decisions ...Decisions!!! If you are sincerely dedicated to living a healthy lifestyle, you can definitely look cute and wear hairstyles conducive to that healthy lifestyle. We shouldn't let our hair prevent us from exercising and being in optimal health. There are many hairstyles that we can wear while keeping up with our fitness goals. Buns, braids, two strand twists and a wide array of

protective styles can be worn while exercising. We can definitely get our workout in and still look super cute. Sooooo……..what do you do with that super cute silk press? Try putting your hair in a tight bun with a cute headband while working out. Wait until your hair totally dries to remove the bun and try pin curling it that night for heatless bouncy curls the next day. This really works ☺.

283. **Sweaty hair issues!** If you are working out regularly and sweat profusely, you may need to cleanse your hair in between workouts. If this is the case for you, try co-washing during the week as needed. As mentioned previously, co-washing is rinsing your hair with water and conditioner. If you shampoo and deep condition weekly and you are working out daily, you may want to co-wash your hair 1-2 times during the week to rinse out the sweat, salt and any buildup that may be present. This will keep your hair and scalp very healthy. It is totally not necessary to shampoo after each and every workout. This will cause dryness which is what you definitely want to avoid.

284. **Try oil rinses.** This is another option for those who exercise daily. The method is super easy. After your sweaty workout, just wet your hair to rinse out the salt and sweat. Then apply a small amount of oil to your hair and scalp. Massage and rinse. Your hair will be very soft and well lubricated. This is one of my favorite ways to refresh my hair after a workout. If you decide to do this method in the shower, be careful not to slip. The oil will make the shower floor super slippery ☺

285. **Swimming and hair damage.** If possible, it is best to seek out a salt water pool because it is chlorine

free which is healthier for your hair and body. If this is not an option, be sure to protect your hair while swimming in a chlorinated pool. Chlorine can be very damaging to the hair and can cause breakage and severe damage. If you protect your hair, you can easily avoid the damage and breakage that chlorine can bring. A great way to protect the hair while swimming is to wet your hair first and then apply oil to the hair before placing on the swim cap. Just think of the hair as being a sponge. If you place a dry sponge in the pool, it will absorb a lot of chlorine. If the sponge is already wet before placing it in the pool, it will absorb very little chlorine. Wetting your hair is like placing a wet sponge in the pool. Minimal chlorine will be absorbed and applying oil will further protect the strands. I swim almost weekly and this is the method that I personally use to prevent damage. This method works like a charm and I have not experienced any breakage.

Product recommendation – Hydratherma Naturals Hair Growth Oil with Emu

286. **Proper cleansing after swimming.** After swimming, be sure to cleanse your hair appropriately to be sure that the chlorine is removed. This is extremely important because you do not want for the chlorine to be left in your hair. This will definitely cause breakage. If you wet your hair and apply oil to your hair before swimming, chlorine absorption should be minimal. The small amount of chlorine left should be easily removed. Product recommendation: Hydratherma Naturals Amino Clarifying Shampoo

HAIR ACCESSORIES

Hair accessories can be downright dangerous if the wrong types are used or if they are used improperly. The improper use of hair accessories can cause breakage and split ends. Hair accessory can also save the day on bad hair days if used correctly. Check out these hair tips below to prevent some of the hair accessory pitfalls.

287. **Stay away from collars, scarves, hats and head wraps made of wool.** As time passes, wool can cause ongoing / slow breakage. If someone is wearing their favorite wool coat daily and their hair goes from mid back length to shoulder length, we know the culprit. Wool can be extremely damaging to the hair and will absolutely cause breakage. Staying away from wool collars, scarves and hats is a good idea if you want to retain length. The constant rubbing of the wool against your hair will surely result in breakage at that particular area (typically the nape area). If you must wear wool, I suggest that you line the inside of the hat and/or collar with a satin scarf. This will cut down on the friction.

288. **Ohhhhhh those bad hair days!** We all know that bad hair days are just a part of life and are to be expected. There is not much that we can do to avoid them. On bad hair days, don't blast your hair with heat. This is the time when you can really experiment with hair accessories like head wraps, clips and styling combs to protective style. Be sure that your hair wraps are not made with fabrics that will break your hair or suck the moisture out. Stay away from 100% cotton and wool. Most other fabrics are safe.

289. **Inspect your hair tools carefully.** Many people overlook this important tip. Before using any hair tool, be sure to inspect it carefully and watch for any sharp edges. Throw away any cracked hair tools that can break off your hair. Splintered rollers and combs with missing teeth are the enemy! Any utensils with sharp ends and rough edges will definitely cause hair breakage so please avoid them.

290. **Rubber bands + loose hair = hair breakage.** If you have loose hair (not loc'd) please don't use rubber bands! Unfortunately, I still know people who are guilty of this travesty. Using rubber bands will absolutely cause tangling (when removed) and will result in breakage. If you do have to use them for some unknown reason, carefully cut them out (to remove them) so that breakage will be avoided. If you have loc'd hair and decide to use rubber bands to hold your braids or twist, it is a bit safer but I still suggest that you carefully cut the rubber bands out of your hair when it is time to remove them.

291. **Examine your ponytail holders.** Stay away from ponytail holders that have metal clips. I still see them being sold at beauty supply stores. The metal potion on the ponytail holder can cause breakage. Instead use ponytail holders that do not contain metal clips to avoid this problem.

292. **Clean your hair accessories frequently.** It is very important to clean your combs, brushes, clippers, scissors and any other hair utensils frequently. This task is often overlooked. Dirty hair utensils are a breeding ground for bacteria and fungi which can cause scalp

infections and ongoing itching. You can disinfect your utensils periodically with biocide or plain alcohol.

293. **Beware of the rat tail comb on wet or dry kinky hair textures if you want to avoid breakage.** In other words, (in most cases) this type of comb should not be used at all to actually comb your hair while in its kinky state. A rat tail comb should only be used for parting the hair (from the pointy end) because it is a very small tooth comb. It can also be used while flat ironing the hair utilizing the chase method. This tip may sound like common sense to most but I have seen people attempt to comb their hair with this small tooth comb numerous times..... I just had to add it to the list ☺

294. **Who loves the old fashioned boar bristle brush?** I remember this brush being a staple in most homes while growing up in the 70's and 80's. We used to slather the hair with water and grease. We then proceeded to use that brush to slick the hair back into a tight ponytail. Lol.......Now that we know better, we have to do better. This particular brush should never be used on wet hair. This will absolutely cause breakage and a thinning hairline. That is why I remember seeing so much hair in these types of brushes while growing up. In my opinion, this brush should be avoided because of its firm bristles. There are many safer options now.

295. **Velcro rollers...Good or bad?** I still see these types of rollers in many beauty supply stores. I actually used to use them back in the 1990's on my short relaxed hair without any problems at first. It was a great heat free method to curl my hair in its straight state but

as time passed, I noticed some problems developing. My hair began to thin so I stopped using them immediately. Many years later, I got my hands on some soft Velcro rollers specifically made for sleeping in. I figured that they would be safe to use because they were soft and flexible. I attempted to use them again on my thick natural hair and it was a disaster. These rollers can wreak havoc on thicker hair textures. I think that velcro rollers can be used safely on straight hair if only used from time to time. If you use them regularly, they will slowly pull the hair out.

296. **Super important bobby pin tip.** PLEASE ......Examine your bobby pins before using them. Many of us just grab a bobby pin and place it in our hair without thinking. I used to be guilty of this. If the bobby pin has a missing bulb on the end, please discard. The sharp tip will cut into the hair strand causing split ends and breakage.

297. Sponge rollers Yay or Nay? Sponge rollers are still a favorite with many because they provide heat free curls and you can sleep in them comfortably due to them being so soft. Many people don't realize that the sponge material is very absorbent and will suck the moisture right out of your hair. The sponge fibers can also snag the hair and cause breakage. There is a solution to this. You can cover the rollers with pieces of satin. There are also sponge rollers that are sold with a satin cover. I actually have some of these satin covered rollers and I absolutely love them. Never use sponge rollers without covering them with satin. You can also use regular white end papers to provide protection.

298. **Remove all styling utensils when retiring to bed.** This includes items such as bobby pins, banana clips, tight ponytail holders and holding combs. These items can rub against your hair scalp while sleeping. This friction will cause breakage, thinning and hair loss.

Warm and Fuzzy Stuff----- Patience, Love and Positive Thinking.

299. **Patience is key!** Have patience on your journey to healthy hair. Be patient and consistent. Stick with your regime and don't give up despite hair "setbacks" that we all go through. Always think of the final goal which is healthy hair. Generally, hair grows ¼ to ½ inch per month. Be persistent and give your hair that extra TLC that it needs. Your hair will love you for it!!!

300. **Love your hair and give it loving / positive energy.** If you love your hair and give it the positive attention that it needs, it will flourish just as a plant would. Your hair may or may not be what you want it to be right now. Love it for what it is now and what it will become in the future. Your hair will definitely respond to your loving energy in a positive way.

301. **Last but not least……..One Bonus Tip!** Think positive! Positive thinking will always lead to positive results. Thinking positive will also attract positive things to you. Frequently look at pictures of your hair inspirations and get excited about the beautiful hair that you will have. Visualize yourself with the hair that you desire. Wake up and speak positive words over your hair such as "I love my hair", "I'm on my way to healthy hair", "My hair is perfect and it is getting better day by day". This may seem silly to some but there is power in positive affirmations. Speak it into existence and it will happen…….only if you believe!

Thanks so much for reading this book. I wrote this book out of my sincere desire to help those having difficulties along their hair journey. I hope that the tips were very helpful to you as you navigate through your healthy hair journey. Please keep in touch with us at info@HealthyHairJourney.com Let us know how your journey is going and send us your progress pictures. We would love to hear from you.

Keep in touch!

xoxo

Website- www.HydrathermaNaturals.com

Facebook www.Facebook.com/Hydratherma

Instagram- www.instagram.com/Hydratherma

Twitter- www.twitter.com/Hydratherma

Email- info@HealthyHairJourney.com

Below are some product recommendations from the Hydratherma Naturals moisture and protein balancing product line that will get your hair healthy and strong.

Hydratherma Naturals Product Recommendations

Moisture Retention

1. Hydratherma Naturals Daily Moisturizing Growth Lotion to moisturize.
2. Hydratherma Naturals Hair Growth Oil to seal in the moisture.
3. Hydratherma Naturals Moisture Boosting Shampoo
4. Hydratherma Naturals Moisture Boosting Conditioning Treatment
5. SLS Free Moisture Plus Hair Cleanser

Protein Boost

1. Hydratherma Naturals Protein Balance Leave In Conditioner
2. Hydratherma Naturals Herbal Amino Clarifying Shampoo
3. Hydratherma Naturals Amino Plus Protein Deep Conditioning Treatment

Natural and Relaxed Hair Stylers for Curl Definition

1. Aloe Curl Enhancing Twisting Cream
2. Foaming Sea Silk Curly Styler
3. Botanical Defining Gel

Scalp Care

1. Hydratherma Naturals Scalp Soothing Shampoo Bar
2. Hydratherma Naturals Hair Growth Oil
3. Hydratherma Naturals Daily Moisturizing Growth Lotion
4. Hydratherma Naturals Follicle Mist

Relaxed Hair Care

1. Hydratherma Naturals Protein Balance Leave In Conditioner
2. Hydratherma Naturals Herbal Amino Clarifying Shampoo
3. Hydratherma Naturals Amino Plus Protein Deep Conditioning Treatment
4. Hydratherma Naturals Daily Moisturizing Growth Lotion to moisturize.
5. Hydratherma Naturals Hair Growth Oil to seal in the moisture.
6. Hydratherma Naturals Moisture Boosting Conditioning Treatment
7. Hydratherma Naturals SLS Free Moisture Plus Hair Cleanser
8. Hydratherma Naturals Foaming Sea Silk Curly Styler
9. Hydratherma Naturals Follicle Mist

Color Treated Hair Care

1. Hydratherma Naturals Protein Balance Leave In Conditioner
2. Hydratherma Naturals Herbal Amino Clarifying Shampoo
3. Hydratherma Naturals Amino Plus Protein Deep Conditioning Treatment
4. Hydratherma Naturals Daily Moisturizing Growth Lotion to moisturize.
5. Hydratherma Naturals Hair Growth Oil to seal in the moisture.

6. Hydratherma Naturals Moisture Boosting Conditioning Treatment
7. SLS Free Moisture Plus Hair Cleanser – Color Safe
8. All stylers

Natural Hair

1. All Hydratherma Naturals Products

Transitioning From Relaxed To Natural

1. All Hydratherma Naturals Products

Protection From Damage

1. Hydratherma Naturals Herbal Gloss Heat Protector
2. Hydratherma Naturals Daily Moisturizing Growth Lotion
3. Hydratherma Naturals Follicle Mist
4. Hydratherma Naturals Hair Growth Oil

All products are available at www.HydrathermaNaturals.com, Amazon and retail locations listed on our website.

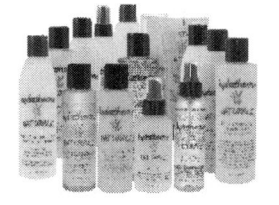

Why the Hydratherma Naturals Healthy Hair Care Product Line Was Created

My time spent as a hair stylist taught me the importance of balancing the moisture and protein levels in the hair. I noticed that when the hair was well balanced, the hair would flourish. Too much moisture or protein would result in breakage. Once the hair was balanced, the hair would thicken, retain length and less breakage would occur. I tried many products on my hair and the hair of my clients. Most products would result in too much moisture in the hair or protein overload. Many clients did not know how to balance the levels in the hair. I wanted to create a line scientifically formulated to balance the moisture and protein levels in the hair. I wanted to take the guess work out of it and make the regimen easy to follow. After several years of combining many of the hair care ingredients that I absolutely loved, we were finally able to formulate a natural-based hair care product collection that left the hair in perfect balance. - Saleemah Cartwright, CEO

This content is for informational purposes only. Information contained in this book is not intended to treat or cure medical conditions or guarantee hair growth. The information is not intended to be a substitute for professional medical advice, diagnosis, treatment or care. Always seek the advice of a medical professional when you have a medical condition. Do not disregard professional medical advice or delay in seeking advice if you have read something in this book. Attempt has been made to verify the information provided in this publication, however, neither the author nor the publisher is responsible for any errors, omissions, or incorrect interpretations of the subject matter. The information provided herein is stated to be truthful and consistent in that, any liability, in terms of inattention or otherwise, by any usage or abuse of any policies, process, or directions contained within is solitary and utter responsibility of the recipient reader. Under no circumstances will any legal responsibility or blame be held against the publisher for any reparation, damages or monetary loss due to the information herein, either directly or indirectly.

Copyright © 2018, Healthy Hair Journey Enterprises, LLC, All Rights Reserved.

Copyright © 2018, Healthy Hair Journey Enterprises, LLC, All Rights Reserved.

No Part of this publication may be reproduced or transmitted in any form or by any means without prior written permission of the copyright holder.

ISBN-13: 978-1986735605
ISBN-10: 1986735605